T0338437

PREVENTION IN NEPHROLOGY

DEVELOPMENTS IN NEPHROLOGY

Volume 28

The Titles published in this series are listed at the end of this volume.

Prevention in nephrology

edited by

MARC E. DE BROE

and

GERT A. VERPOOTEN
University Hospital Antwerp, Edegem, Belgium

Kluwer Academic Publishers
Dordrecht / Boston / London

Library of Congress Cataloging-in-Publication Data

```
Prevention in nephrology / edited by Marc E. de Broe, Gert A.
  Verpooten.
      p.   cm. -- (Developments in nephrology ; 28)
  Includes bibliographical references.
  Includes index.
  ISBN 0-7923-0951-0 (HB : alk. paper)
  1. Kidneys--Diseases--Prevention.   I. De Broe, M. E. (Marc E.)
II. Verpooten, Gert A.   III. Series.
  [DNLM: 1. Kidney Diseases--prevention & control.   W1 DE998EB v.
28 / WJ 300 P9435]
RC903.P7  1991
616.6'105--dc20
DNLM/DLC
for Library of Congress                                  90-5202
```

ISBN 0-7923-0951-0

Published by Kluwer Academic Publishers,
P.O. Box 17, 3300 AA Dordrecht, The Netherlands.

Kluwer Academic Publishers incorporates
the publishing programmes of
D. Reidel, Martinus Nijhoff, Dr W. Junk and MTP Press.

Sold and distributed in the U.S.A. and Canada
by Kluwer Academic Publishers,
101 Philip Drive, Norwell, MA 02061, U.S.A.

In all other countries, sold and distributed
by Kluwer Academic Publishers Group,
P.O. Box 322, 3300 AH Dordrecht, The Netherlands.

Printed on acid-free paper

Printed in The Netherlands

Contents

List of major contributors

C. Amiel, Université Paris VII, Inserm U 251, Faculté de Médecine Xavier Bichat, Laboratoire de Physiologie Rénale, 16, rue Henri Huchard, F-75018 Paris, France

J.C. Christiansen, Second University Clinic of Internal Medicine (diabetes and endocrinology), Kommunehospital, DK-8000 Aarhus, Denmark

M.E. de Broe, Department of Nephrology-Hypertension, University Hospital Antwerp, Wilrijkstraat 10, B-2520, Edegem, Belgium.

J.P. Deslypere, Department of Endocrinology, University Hospital, De Pintelaan 185, B-9000 Gent, Belgium

U.C. Dubach, Medizinische Universitätspoliklinik, Abt. Innere Med., Kantonsspital, Petersgraben 4, CH-4031 Basel, Switzerland

J.P. Grünfeld, Hôpital Necker, Département de Néphrologie, 161, rue de Sèvres, F-75730 Paris Cedex 15, France

H.H. Malluche, University of Kentucky, Department of Nephrology, (bone and mineral metabolism), Room MN572, Lexington, KY 40536-0084, U.S.A.

H. Mattie, Department of Infectious Diseases, University Hospital Leiden, Bldg. 1, C5-P, P.O. Box 9600, NL-2300 RC Leiden, The Netherlands

B.M. Tune, Stanford University School of Medicine, Division of Pediatric Nephrology, Stanford, CA 94305-5119, U.S.A.

G.A. Verpooten, Department of Nephrology-Hypertension, University Hospital Antwerp, Wilrijkstraat 10, B-2520, Edegem, Belgium.

R.P. Wedeen, U.S. Department of Veteran Affairs, Medical Center, Tremont Avenue, East Orange, NJ 07019, U.S.A.

J.J. Weening, University of Groningen, Department of Pathology, Oostersingel 63, NL-9713 EZ Groningen, The Netherlands

Prevention of renal disease: An overview

J.P. GRÜNFELD

Prevention of disease is one of the primary goals of medicine. The rapid escalation of the cost of medical care during the past three decades has highlighted but was not at the origin of the need for prevention. Prevention is difficult in diseases in which several deleterious factors are involved, and where the pathogenesis and pathophysiology have not been clarified. Prevention and research are closely associated.

Prevention may be schematically subdivided into "primary" (to prevent the appearance of diseases) and "secondary" (to reduce the rate of progression and the complications of diseases). Both these approaches have been used in nephrology and will be illustrated later in this book. My aim is not to cover the whole field of prevention in nephrology, but rather to focus on some issues that show what can be done and what are the future challenges in the prevention of renal disease. I will not deal with "tertiary" prevention (prevention of the consequences of hypertension, of bone uremic disease, etc.) which has been successfully developed in recent decades. More complete information on prevention of kidney and urinary tract diseases can be found elsewhere [1, 2].

1. In recent decades, primary prevention has been achieved in some renal diseases

The most striking example of recently acquired prevention is in acute renal failure in pregnancy. In the 1950s and 1960s, as many as 22% of all cases of acute renal failure were obstetric in origin, with mortality rates ranging from 16 to 48%, where today renal failure occurs in less than 1% of all pregnancies in Western countries [3]. Concordant data have been collected in Dublin, Paris, Chicago, Birmingham (England), and Leeds [4]. Con-

M. E. De Broe and G. A. Verpooten (eds.): Prevention in Nephrology, 1–8.
© 1991 *Kluwer Academic Publishers. Printed in the Netherlands.*

comitantly, the incidence of bilateral cortical necrosis in pregnant women declined dramatically [3].

Several factors have contributed to the decline in pregnancy-related acute renal failure, such as the disappearance or sharp decrease in septic abortions, improvement in obstetric care, and more successful early intervention in the management of complicated pregnancy. This progress is well illustrated in the recent study by Turney *et al.* [4]: during the period 1960–64, obstetric hemorrhage was the triggering factor in 30% of the cases of acute renal failure, whereas in the 1970–87 period, it represented only approximately 10% of the causes. Preeclampsia-related acute renal failure accounted for 80% of the cases in the latter period, and it is well known that this cause leads to relatively benign acute renal failure [3]. In contrast, in less developed countries, the incidence of pregnancy-induced acute renal failure remains high [3].

In recent decades, the incidence of membranoproliferative glomerulonephritis has decreased strikingly in Western European countries. This has been well demonstrated in France, Italy, and Spain [5, 6]. The explanations for this phenomenon are still obscure. More adequate control of seasonal infections might play a role. It is surprising to see how unplanned prevention may work. The identification of the underlying mechanism is, however, of great interest for understanding the pathogenesis of some glomerular diseases. The lessons gained from prevention may generate hypotheses concerning pathogenesis. In addition, good epidemiological data are necessary in order to consider and to assess preventive measures. This statement is illustrated in other chapters of this book.

2. In many instances, prevention lies beyond nephrology

Some examples are listed in Table I. In this regard, there is no "preventive nephrology" but there is preventive medicine, a part of which is devoted to renal diseases. These examples also show that good circulation of information plays a key role in prevention, and this information should be directed to the general population, nurses, social workers, and doctors, general practitioners or specialists in various fields. Nephrologists should be well aware that prevention of some renal diseases necessitates close collaboration with these various groups.

Table I. Examples showing that prevention lies beyond nephrology

Primary goal (beyond nephrology)	Ultimate goal (within nephrology)
To prevent or arrest abusive analgesic consumption	To prevent nephropathy due to analgesic abuse
Adequate management of diabetes mellitus (including blood pressure control)	To prevent diabetic nephropathy
Adequate use of potentially nephrotoxic drugs	To prevent drug-induced nephrotoxicity
Early detection of urinary tract infection in children	To detect and manage urinary tract malformations, and prevent renal scars
Less aggressive surgery and rational use of non-surgical means in nephrolithiasis	To prevent stone-induced chronic pyelonephritis
Identification and eradication of lead intoxication	To prevent lead nephrotoxicity
Colchicine therapy in familial Mediterranean fever	To prevent renal amyloidosis

3. Prevention in nephrology rests in part on identifying high-risk groups and targeting preventive measures toward them

Prevention of most renal diseases should be aimed at high-risk patients, whereas prevention of some other diseases, such as essential hypertension, may apply to the general population. The results of systematic screening for proteinuria or microhematuria in young adults are not rewarding. In contrast, dipstick screening for hematuria might be useful in subjects over 50 or 60 years, particularly men, to detect urological malignancy [7], although this procedure should be tested in a population-based controlled trial [7, 8]. The main problem is therefore to *identify high-risk groups.* Current possibilities and difficulties are illustrated in the following examples:

3.1. Pregnancy-related renal complications

The prevention of acute pyelonephritis in pregnancy is based, in large part, on the early detection and treatment of asymptomatic bacteriuria, whose prevalence ranges between 2 and 10%. Higher rates have been observed in multiparous women from low socioeconomic classes [2], and in pregnant women with a history of recurrent urinary tract infection, sickle cell trait or diabetes. However, detection and therapy of asymptomatic bacteriuria appears to prevent only 50 to 70% of potential antepartum pyelonephritis [9]. Many authors advocate routine screening for bacteriuria in all gravidas at their initial prenatal visit, in the first trimester, whereas others suggest that testing be limited to high-risk women.

Several recent trials have shown that administration of aspirin, at various doses, alone or in association with dipyridamole exerted a preventive effect against preeclampsia [10–12]. The inclusion criteria are different in these three randomized controlled studies (Table II). High-risk women have been defined as follows: nulliparous or primagravidae, twin gestation, history of preeclampsia or fetal death, increased blood pressure response to i.v. infusion of angiotensin II and/or positive rollover test at 28–29 weeks of gestation. In all these three trials (including relatively small numbers of gravidas), striking prevention of preeclampsia was achieved in actively treated women. Larger-scale clinical trials are in progress or have been completed in France and the U.S. to confirm the efficacy, safety, scope and modalities of this therapy in relatively high-risk women.

Table II. Prospective trials with antiplatelet agents showing prevention of preeclampsia

	Inclusion criteria	Active treatment	
		Start	Doses
Beaufils *et al.*	High risk of preeclampsia and/or fetal retardation	12 weeks of gestation	150 mg aspirin + 300 mg dipyridamole/day
Wallenburg *et al.*	Primigravidae + increased blood pressure response to i.v. angiotensin II	28 weeks of gestation	100 mg aspirin/day
Schiff *et al.*	Nulliparity, twin gestation or history of preeclampsia + positive rollover test at 28–29 weeks	28–29 weeks of gestation	60 mg aspirin/day

3.2. Nephrosclerosis

Nephrosclerosis, as a renal consequence of severe or malignant hypertension, accounts for 15 to 20% of all cases of renal failure in the United States. Renal failure due to hypertension is 15 to 18 times more frequent in blacks than in whites (see the references in [13]).

It is still controversial whether this predisposition depends on genetic factors, socioeconomic factors [14] or both. In addition, the high prevalence of non-insulin dependent diabetes mellitus in blacks may accelerate the development of renal vascular changes [15]. Abnormally low preglomerular vascular resistance may expose glomerular capillaries more directly to the deleterious effect of elevated blood pressure. Such an abnormality might be suggested from the data presented by Luft *et al.* showing higher creatinine clearance in young blacks and more rapid deterioration with aging than in whites [16]. Whatever the pathophysiologic explanation, the efforts toward preventing nephrosclerosis should be aimed at better detection and control of hypertension, in blacks and probably in all subjects of low socioeconomic and educational levels. However, Rostand *et al.* have indicated that, surprisingly, deterioration of renal function may develop in some patients despite good blood pressure control, and this occurs most particularly in black patients [16].

3.3. Diabetes mellitus

Prevention of diabetic nephropathy is discussed by Mogensen *et al.* in this volume. Recent studies have identified diabetic patients at high risk of nephropathy (see the references in [17]), i.e. patients with poor glycemic control, patients with a familial predisposition to hypertension and with an overactive sodium-lithium exchange system in red blood cells, patients with a family history of diabetic nephropathy, black patients with non-insulin-dependent diabetes, and possibly males and smokers. Careful management and monitoring may be mandatory in these patients, although the value of some of these predisposing factors has been challenged. In addition, prevention of insulin-dependent diabetes itself in high-risk families may be considered. Autoimmune disorders precede complete destruction of pancreatic beta cells, and adequate and early intervention may be expected in the future.

3.4. Inherited kidney disease

Identification of high-risk patients is also of great interest in inherited kidney diseases since they are clinically and genetically heterogeneous. Autosomal dominant polycystic kidney disease (ADPKD) is an example of this heterogeneity. In some patients and in some families, ADPKD is associated with cerebral artery aneurysms. It is crucial to detect these high-risk families (or patients) before rupture of the berry aneurysms. No genetic marker for berry aneurysm is so far available, and no investigational protocol has been prospectively tested. The rate of progression to renal failure is also heterogeneous in ADPKD [18]. Two epidemiological studies have shown that for ADPKD patients, the probability of being alive and not having end-stage renal failure by the age of 50 years if 77 and 78% respectively. By the age of 73 years, this probability is still high, at 52%. No marker is known for early identification of the ADPKD at higher risk of progression. If markers were available, more careful monitoring and earlier intervention would be justified in these patients to delay or to prevent end-stage renal disease. A cooperative European study is in progress in this regard.

Obviously, the progress in molecular genetics has raised the possibility of prenatal diagnosis. This has been applied to ADPKD, in the forms linked to the PKD1 locus, on the short arm of chromosome 16. Great caution should be exercised against indiscriminate use of prenatal diagnosis in ADPKD families [21]. In brief, the mutant gene itself has not so far been identified and directly studied; linkage study does not provide information on the rate of progression, and the ethical basis for prenatal diagnosis and interruption of pregnancy has been questioned.

3.5. Primary glomerulonephritis

Little attention has been focussed on risk factors in primary glomerulonephritis. In Berger's disease, male sex is recognized in all series as indicative of risk of progression. Similarly, in membranous nephropathy, male sex and the presence and persistence of the nephrotic syndrome are associated with poor renal prognosis. Early control of slight hypertension is probably of crucial importance in these high-risk groups. A decrease in blood pressure might also be desirable, even in high-risk normotensive patients. In addition, prospective therapeutic trials should in the future focus on these high-risk groups.

References

1. Coggins CH, Cummings NB (eds), 1978: *Prevention of Kidney and Urinary Tract Diseases*, DHEW Pub. No. (NIH) 78–855, p. 297.
2. Grünfeld JP, Legrain S, 1979: Quelles maladies rénales peut-on prévenir?, in *Actualités Néphrologiques de l'Hôpital Necker*. Hamburger J, Crosnier J and Funck-Brentano J-L (eds), Flammarion, Paris.
3. Pertuiset N, Grünfeld JP, 1987: Acute renal failure in pregnancy, in *Renal Disease in Pregnancy*. Lindheimer MD and Davison JM (eds), Ballière Tindall, London, pp. 873–90.
4. Turney JH, Ellis CM, Parsons FM, 1989: Obstetric acute renal failure 1956–1987. Br J Obstet Gyn 96: 679–87.
5. Jungers P, Droz D, Noël LH, Fétizon D, Manganella J, Grünfeld JP, 1982: Is membranoproliferative glomerulonephritis (MPGN) disappearing in France? Kidney Int 21: 899.
6. Jungers P, Forget D, Droz D, Noël LH, Grünfeld JP, 1985: Membranoproliferative glomerulonephritis (MPGN) is disappearing in France: Epidemiologic data on 1231 patients with primary chronic glomerulonephritis. Kidney Int 27: 829.
7. Britton JP, Dowell AC, Whelan P, 1989: Dipstick haematuria and bladder cancer in men over 60: results of a community study. Br Med J 299: 1010–2.
8. Woolhandler S, Pels RJ, Bor DH, Himmelstein DU, Lawrence RS, 1989: Dipstick urinalysis screening of asymptomatic adults for urinary tract disorders. JAMA 262: 1215–20.
9. Lawson DH, Miller AWF, 1973: Screening for bacteriuria in pregnancy. A critical appraisal. Arch intern Med 132: 904.
10. Beaufils M, Uzan S, Donsimoni R, Colau JC, 1985: Prevention of pre-eclampsia by early antiplatelet therapy. Lancet 1: 840–2.
11. Wallenburg HCS, Dekker GA, Makovitz JW, Rotmans P, 1986: Low-dose aspirin prevents pregnancy-induced hypertension and pre-eclampsia in angiotensin-sensitive primigravidae. Lancet 1: 8471–3.
12. Schiff E, Peleg E, Goldenberg M, *et al.*, 1989: The use of aspirin to prevent pregnancy-induced hypertension and lower the ratio of thromboxane A_2 to prostacyclin in relatively high risk pregnancies. N Engl J Med 321: 351–6.
13. Rostand SG, Brown G, Kirk KA, Rutsky EA, Dustan HP, 1989: Renal insufficiency in treated essential hypertension. N Engl J Med 320: 684–8.
14. Ooi WL, Budner NS, Cohen H, Madhavan S, Alderman MH, 1989: Impact of race on treatment response and cardiovascular disease among hypertensives. Hypertension 14: 227:34.
15. Tierney WM, McDonald CJ, Luft FC, 1989: Renal disease in hypertensive adults: Effect of race and type II diabetes mellitus. Am J Kidney Dis. 13: 485–93.
16. Luft FC, Fineberg NS, Miller JZ *et al.*, 1980: The effects of age, race, and heredity on glomerular filtration rate following volume expansion and contraction in normal man. Am J Med Sci 279: 15–24.
17. Seaquist ER, Goetz FC, Rich S, Barbosa J, 1989: Familial clustering of diabetic kidney disease. Evidence for genetic susceptibility to diabetic nephropathy. N Engl J Med 320: 1161–5.

8

18. Grünfeld JP, Noël LH, Bobrie G, *et al.* 19XX: Advances in the understanding of inherited renal diseases, in *Nephrology* Vol I, Davison AM (ed). Baillière Tindall, London, pp. 637–60.

Evaluation and significance of renal functional reserve in health and disease

CLAUDE AMIEL, FRANÇOISE BLANCHET,
GÉRARD FRIEDLANDER, & ALAIN NITENBERG

The term *renal functional reserve* appeared for the first time, to the best of our knowledge, in a publication by Bosch *et al.* [1] where it was defined as "... the ability of the kidney to increase its level of operation under certain demands".

Common usage of the concept limits the level of operation to the glomerular filtration rate (GFR) and the renal plasma flow (RPF), thus excluding all situations where tubular functions are challenged.

Several situations are known to involve an increase in GFR and RPF: protein load and amino acid infusion, pregnancy, compensatory renal hypertrophy, burns, and diabetes. Such knowledge is not recent. Pitts [2] wrote, in 1944,

> ... intravenous administration of the amino acid glycin duplicates rapidly and reversibly those changes in the renal circulation which are seen over a period of hours following a protein meal, and permits the ready investigation of the changes in renal tone which serve as their basis.

Undoubtedly, the recent interest for the RFR arose from the hypothesis formulated by the Brenner group [3–5] of detrimental effects of hyperfiltration:

> We are intrigued by the possibility that augmented intrarenal pressures and flows associated with *ad libitum* feeding contribute to the age-associated glomerular sclerosis repeatedly observed in laboratory animals,

and

> The biologic price of the adaptation to *ad libitum* feeding is acceptable in the absence of diabetes, acquired renal diseases, or surgical loss of renal mass. But the more pronounced elevations in glomerular pressure and flow associated with these latter conditions may accelerate the develop-

M. E. De Broe and G. A. Verpooten (eds.): Prevention in Nephrology, 9–23.
© 1991 *Kluwer Academic Publishers. Printed in the Netherlands.*

ment of glomerular sclerosis, leading to more rapid loss of renal function.

In this short review, the following aspects of the RFR will be examined:

1. Evaluation of the RFR
2. Mechanisms which bring into play the RFR
3. The RFR in disease
4. What can be expected from the determination of the RFR?

1. Evaluation of the RFR: Maneuvers which increase RPF and GFR

Several maneuvers are known to increase RPF and GFR: oral protein load, amino acid infusion, glucagon infusion, dopamine infusion.

1.1. An oral protein load was used by Pitts in 1944, by Pullman *et al.* in 1954 and by O'Connor and Summerill in 1976 [2, 6, 7]. Since then, Bosch *et al.* [1, 8, 9] have repeatedly utilized this stimulus, administering 70–80 g of protein in the form of cooked red meat over 30 min. The peak values of RPF and GFR were obtained after 1 to 2 hr. Similarly, Hostetter [10] employed lean cooked beef steak, 3.5 g/kg of b.w.

1.2. Amino acids infusion has been used, since the already mentioned pioneer work of Pitts [2], by many authors (see [11–23]). The rate of administration varied between 1 and 8 mg/kg/min and the duration of the infusion between 45 min and 18 hr. Peak values of RPF and GFR were observed between 15 to 180 min after starting the infusion. Most authors used mixtures of amino acids, although several, including Pitts [2], used individual amino acids (alanine, arginine, glycine). Branched-chain aminoacid infusion does not induce any increase in RPF and GFR [24].

1.3. Since the work of Levy and Starr [25] it has become known that glucagon infusion increases RPF and GFR. This was confirmed by many authors [11, 15, 19, 21, 26–31]. The lowest rate of infusion to man was 4 ng/kg/min.

1.4. Practical determination of RFR can be achieved with any of the three stimuli mentioned above. The difficulty is obtaining a reliable determination of GFR, which implies that polyfructosan clearance should be preferred to creatinine clearance. Polyfructosan and paraaminohippurate clearance measurements (the latter in order to estimate RPF) can be obtained before and after the exposure to the stimulus. Water load is useful to ensure a large urinary output in order to minimize the errors linked to incomplete bladder voiding.

2. Mechanisms which bring into play the RFR

The main mechanisms which have been thought to play a role in the elicitation of RFR are alteration of tubuloglomerular feedback, modification of angiotensin circulating concentration, growth hormone or other hypophyseal hormone releases, glucagon release, and prostaglandins synthesis.

2.1. Alteration of tubuloglomerular feedback

It was well demonstrated by Seney and Wright [32] that during the administration of a high protein diet to rats, the activity of the tubuloglomerular feedback was decreased. The difference between SNGFRs measured in a proximal tubule and in a distal tubule of the same nephron was significantly smaller than under controls, whereas the loop perfusion rate, which could elicit a half-maximal decrease of stop-flow pressure, was significantly larger than during controls. Similarly, Woods et al. [33] concluded from a study on dogs that aminoacid infusion induced hyperfiltration through an alteration of tubuloglomerular feedback. Seney et al. [34] further demonstrated that the decreased activity of tubuloglomerular feedback was accounted for by a lower signal at the macula densa, a consequence of an increased reabsorption of sodium and chloride in the thick ascending limb of Henle. Finally, Bouby et al. [35] showed that a high protein diet could induce an hypertrophy of the ascending limb, thus providing a structural explanation for the increased reabsorption of sodium and chloride. However important those latter findings are, it is unlikely that they account for the increase in RPF and GFR observed within minutes after the ingestion of a protein load or the infusion of aminoacids.

2.2. Angiotensin II

Ruilope et al. [22] obtained, in man, results indicating that a low Na diet could prevent the renal vasodilatory effects of aminoacids and that converting enzyme inhibition restored, during a low Na diet, the renal hemodynamic effects of aminoacids. They concluded that an excess of angiotensin II could blunt the hemodynamic response to aminoacids. At variance, Corman et al. [36], using rats as a model, showed that the inhibition of converting enzymes resulted in blunting the increase in GFR produced by a protein-rich diet. Finally, Paller and Hostetter [37] concluded from a study of the effects of a 10 day, protein-rich diet, the effects of which included increased plasma renin activity and increased pressor responsiveness to angiotensin II, that the primary effect of the diet could have been an increased prostaglandin synthesis.

2.3. Growth hormone

The possible role of growth hormone (GH) in the increase of RPF and GFR relies on a series of observation: (i) It was shown that GH increased rapidly and transiently after an aminoacid load [38]; (ii) GH administration increased RPF and GFR [39, 40]; (iii) Acromegaly was associated with high RPF and GFR [41]; and (iv) aminoacids failed to increase GFR in HG deficient patients and in patients with hypophyseal hormone deficiencies [42].

There is, however, contrary evidence that Plasma GH did not correlate with GPR during aminoacid infusion [18] and aminoacids increased RPF and GFR in six GH-deficient patients [20]. Finally, it was shown by Hirschberg et al. [43] that the GH-induced, late increase in GFR was accounted for by a similarly late augmented release of IGF1. Indeed, IGF1 infusion was shown to increase GFR and RPF in rats, an effect which was blocked by indomethacin but not by somatostatin [44].

2.4. Glucagon

2.4.1. The involvement of glucagon in the RFR can be derived from four groups of facts:
  (i)   The administration of aminoacids stimulated glucagon release as repeatedly shown in [45–49];
  (ii) Exogenous glucagon could mimick the renal hemodynamic effects of aminoacids [11, 15, 19, 21, 23, 25–31];
  (iii) A blockade of endogenous glucagon release by somatostatin prevented the aminoacid-induced increase of RPF and GFR [14, 15, 18, 19, 23, 31];

(iv) Aminoacid infusion failed to increase RPF and GFR in six pancreatectomized patients, whereas exogenous glucagon increased GFR [23]. Bergstrom *et al.* [50], however, challenged the role of glucagon because, in their observations, the increase in GFR preceded that of the plasma glucagon concentration. Premen *et al.* [31] challenged the role of glucagon on the grounds that the increase in plasma glucagon observed in dogs after a protein-rich meal was not able, when reproduced by an infusion of exogenous glucagon, to induce similar renal hemodynamic changes. However, it is likely that similar systemic glucagonemias do not reflect a similar portal glucagon concentration during glucagon infusion, on the one hand, and protein ingestion, on the other. Indeed, the portal-peripheral gradient was shown to increase markedly during the stimulation of glucagon release, as in aminoacid infusion [51].

2.4.2. The mechanism of the effect of glucagon is still unknown. A direct effect on the renal vasculature was suggested by results obtained by Okamura *et al.* [52] showing that the hormone induced the relaxation of isolated renal arteries, probably through cAMP generation. A similar conclusion was reached from in-vivo studies by Johannesen *et al.* [11]. However, glucagon infused in the renal artery did not alter RPF and GFR in dogs [30] or in man [23]. An indirect effect is therefore likely. This effect was shown to be independent of the release of glucose in the circulation [53].

The role of the liver was suggested by several observations (for review, see [54, 55]): (i) Portal infusion of aminoacids [56] but not infusion in the renal artery (see above) induced renal vasodilation; (ii) Aminoacid infusion did not affect the GFR of patients with impaired hepatic function [57]; and (iii) glucagon was ineffective in increasing the GFR in dogs with experimental cirrhosis and ascites [58]. The role of the liver, however, was negated by Woods *et al.* [59].

Regarding the possible role of the liver, the Uranga group [56, 60–63] postulated the existence of a renal vasodilator agent which they called *glomerulopressin*. In a similar approach, Zimmerman *et al.* [64] isolated a factor from venous liver blood, identified with serotonin, which increased the contractile tension of gastric strips and the concentration of which increased when liver blood was collected after the intragastric infusion of aminoacids. Finally, it should be mentioned that glucagon could also act through an alteration of tubuloglomerular feedback because it may increase

Na and Cl reabsorption in the thick ascending limb [28]. This effect, however, lacks experimental assessment in man.

2.5. Prostaglandins

That prostaglandins are a mediator of protein or aminoacid increase in RPF and GFR has been repeatedly demonstrated: Levine et al. [65] showed that the inhibition of prostaglandin synthesis prevented the hemodynamic effects of an albumin load in rats and Ruilope et al. [23], Hirschberg et al. [22], and Vanrenterghem et al. [66] showed that prostaglandin synthesis inhibition prevented the hemodynamic effects of aminoacid infusion in man. At variance with those results, Benigni et al. [67] reported that indomethacin inhibited urinary excretion of vasodilatory prostaglandins but did not prevent hyperfiltration in normal rats fed a high-protein diet.

The role of prostaglandins was located by Hirschberg et al. [21] beyond the glucagon release, inasmuch as the inhibition of prostaglandin synthesis prevented a glucagon-induced rise in RPF and GFR. As mentioned above, prostaglandins appear to be instrumental in the vasodilatory effect of IGF1 as well. Furthermore, it was shown that the PGE2 and PGF1 alpha synthetic rate by isolated rat glomeruli was increased when the glomeruli were obtained from protein loaded rats [65, 68].

Finally, interactions are possible between prostaglandins and serotonin, inasmuch as serotonin stimulates PGE2 and prostacyclin synthesis in mesangial cells [69] and the inhibition of PG synthesis reverses the serotonin-induced renal vasodilation into sustained vasoconstriction [70].

2.6. Multifactorial effect

The determinism of hemodynamic changes may actually involve other factors. Indeed, Castellino et al. [71] concluded, from a study of dogs, that the increase in RPF and GFR necessitated the simultaneous existence of hyperaminoacidemia and of increased circulating concentrations of GH, glucagon, and insulin.

2.7. Hypothetic cascade of events linking protein ingestion or aminoacid infusion and increase in RPF and GFR

Figure 1 indicates the steps of a hypothetic, and most likely erroneous, cascade of events linking protein ingestion or aminoacid infusion and an increase in RPF and GFR. Protein ingestion or aminoacid infusion induces glucagon release by the pancreas and stimulates glomerular synthesis of vasodilatory prostaglandins. Glucagon would induce the release by the liver of a vasodilatory factor, possibly serotonin, which would act both by further stimulating the glomerular synthesis of vasodilatory protaglandins and by a direct renal vasodilatory action.

HYPOTHETIC CASCADE OF EVENTS LINKING PROTEIN INGESTION OR AMINO ACID INFUSION AND INCREASE IN RPF AND GFR

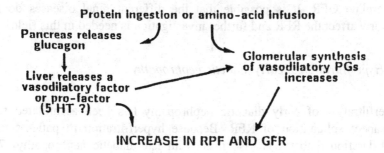

Fig. 1.

3. The renal reserve in disease

The following three items will now be discussed:

Evolution of the RFR when baseline GFR is decreasing as a consequence of kidney disease;
Diabetic hyperfiltration;
Hyperfiltration and progression of renal failure.

3.1. Evolution of the RFR when baseline GFR is decreasing as a consequence of kidney disease

There are three theoretical possibilities about the pattern of RFR evolution when GFR decreases. The first is that the RFR decreases progressively to zero before any diminution of baseline RFR, the second is a decrease of RFR in proportion to the decrease of baseline GFR, i.e. that RFR would be a constant fraction of baseline GFR, and the third is that RFR decreases proportionally more than GFR, thus reaching a zero value at some decreased value of baseline GFR. Data collected in [1, 8–10, 16–19, 21, 22, 72–75] and representing values obtained from healthy subjects, subjects with a solitary kidney or a remnant kidney after donation of the opposite, subjects with a transplanted kidney, and subjects with renal diseases, seem to favor the third possibility. The RFR would be annihilated for values of GFR below 50–70 ml/min. Results obtained from experimental models, however, are at variance: Kleinknecht *et al.* (personal communication) observed in rats with renal mass reduction that RFR was a constant fraction of baseline GFR. It is possible that the different renal diseases do not similarly affect the RFR and further investigation is needed in this field.

3.2. Hyperfiltration of early diabetic nephropathy

Hyperfiltration of early diabetic nephropathy has been assimilated to a permanent solicitation of RFR. Because hyperfiltration in patients with short-duration diabetes is associated with late-diabetic nephropathy [76], considerable interest has been devoted to studies of mechanisms possibly involved in hyperfiltration of diabetes (for a review, see [77]). Those possible mechanisms are:

Hyperglycemia;
Increased circulating levels of glucagon;
Increased renal synthesis of prostaglandins;
Increased circulating levels of atrial natriuretic peptide;
Increased protein uptake;
Renal enlargement.

3.2.1. Hyperglycemia was shown to be a contributive factor that could worsen the hyperfiltration [78–79]. Woods *et al.* [80], using an animal model, showed that hyperglycemia impaired autoregulation and increased RPF and GFR through a tubuloglomerular feedback mechanism triggered by a decreased delivery of sodium to the macula densa, itself resulting from an increased sodium proximal reabsorption induced by the augmented glucose load to the sodium-glucose cotransport.

3.2.2. Different opinions were expressed as to the role of elevated circulating levels of glucagon and GH in diabetic hyperfiltration. A study by Parving *et al.* [81] concluded that glucagon and GH contributed to hyperfiltration only in poorly regulated diabetics but not in well controlled ones. Along the same lines, Wiseman *et al.* [82] concluded that elevated plasma concentration of glucagon and GH did not characterize hyperfiltering diabetic patients. Hostetter *et al.* [5], however, observed that augmented levels of glucagon and GH are common in diabetic hyperglycemia and may contribute to hyperfiltration.

3.2.3. Increased renal synthesis of prostaglandins by glomeruli of diabetic rats was demonstrated [83, 84], thereby suggesting that vasodilatory prostaglandins may play a critical role in the diabetic hyperfiltration.

3.2.4. Ortola *et al.* [85] demonstrated increased circulating levels of atrial natriuretic peptide in diabetic rats which could explain the hyperfiltration. The increased release of the peptide could be secondary to extracellular fluid volume expansion caused by increased sodium proximal reabsorption induced by the augmented glucose load to the sodium-glucose cotransport.

3.2.5. Increased protein uptake by diabetics was considered by Kupin *et al.* [86] as a possible determinant of hyperfiltration inasmuch as the restriction of protein intake to the same level as in healthy controls, blunted hyperfiltration.

3.2.6. Hirose *et al.* [87] and Ellis *et al.* [88] suggested that the renal enlargement observed in diabetic patients could account for the hyperfiltration because of the increase in filtration area. Wiseman *et al.* [78], however, obtained normalization of GFR by strict glycemic control, despite the persistent enlargement of the kidneys.

3.3. Hyperfiltration and progression of renal failure

The available data, briefly reviewed here, raise two questions: Is hyperfiltration a detrimental factor responsible for the progression of renal failure?; Is the beneficial effect of protein restriction exerted through diminished hyperfiltration?

As mentioned above, it is the proposal of the Brenner and Hostetter groups that a sustained increase in plasma flow and SNGFR, together with increased glomerular pressure, results in damaging remnant glomeruli. This proposal has had a tremendous stimulating effect on the analysis of the mechanisms of the progression of renal disease. One should be aware, however, that it has not been established that increased plasma flow, SNGFR, and glomerular pressure are obligatory intermediates of glomerular damage.

There are at least two experimental circumstances where other mechanisms are involved: Yoshida et al. [89] demonstrated very elegantly in a remnant model of rats that the degree of hyperfiltration did not correlate with the extent of subsequent structural damage. Bertani et al. [90] and Grond et al. [91] observed that puromycin and adriamycin-induced nephrosis could lead to glomerulosclerosis without any increase in SNGFR or intraglomerular pressure. Finally, that hyperfiltration does not necessarily lead to glomerular damage was suggested by the absence of proven deterioration of the remnant hypertrophied kidney in subjects who have donated the opposite kidney [74].

In several models of experimental renal disease, protein restriction blunts hyperfiltration and reduces the progression of renal injury. The mechanism by which protein restriction slowed the deterioration of renal function was claimed to be a decrease in glomerular capillary hydraulic pressure [92]. The possible existence of mechanisms of progression of renal damage other than an increase in SNGFR or glomerular pressure, suggests that protein restriction may also act through other pathways.

From the above-mentioned data, it results that the identification of the factors responsible for the progression of renal disease remains a timely topic which deserves further experimental work and clinical investigation.

4. What can be expected from the determination of RFR?

4.1. RFR is not an index of remnant renal tissue. As indicated above, RFR may be a constant fraction of GFR, or it may decrease more rapidly than GFR. In both cases, RFR cannot be considered as the index of remnant renal tissue which would be so useful in the evaluation of the diseased kidney.

4.2. If one accepts the hypothesis that hyperfiltration is detrimental for the remnant renal tissue, one may want to give the low protein diet which is concomitant with the larger RFR, i.e. the least hyperfiltration [93].

4.3. Further clinical investigation, conducted along rigorous prospective protocols, is necessary to document the pattern of alteration of the RFR in different nephropathies and different nephrotoxic aggressions.

References

1. Bosch JP, Saccaggi A, Lauer A, Ronco C, Belledonne M, Glabman S, 1983: Renal functional reserve in humans. Effect of protein intake on glomerular filtration rate. Am J Med 75: 943–50.
2. Pitts RF, 1944: The effects of infusing glycin and of varying the dietary protein intake on renal hemodynamics in the dog. Am J Physiol 142: 355–65.
3. Hostetter TH, Olson JL, Rennke HG, Venkatachalam MA, Brenner BM, 1981: Hyperfiltration in remnant nephrons: A potentially adverse response to renal ablation. Am J Physiol 241: F85–F93.
4. Brenner BM, Meyer TW, Hostetter TH, 1982: Dietary protein intake and the progressive nature of kidney disease: The role of hemodynamically mediated glomerular injury in the pathogenesis of progressive glomerular sclerosis in aging, renal ablation, and intrinsic renal disease. New Engl J Med 307: 652–9.
5. Hostetter TH, Rennke HG, Brenner BM, 1982: The case for intrarenal hypertension in the initiation and progression of diabetic and other glomerulopathies. Am J Med 72: 375–80.
6. Pullman TN, Alving AS, Dern RJ, Landowne M, 1954: The influence of dietary protein intake on specific renal functions in normal man. J Lab Clin Invest 44: 320–32.
7. O'Connor WJ, Summerill RA, 1976: The effect of a meal of meat on glomerular filtration rate in dogs at normal urine flows. J Physiol 256: 81–91.
8. Bosch JP, Lauer A, Glabman S, 1984: Short-term protein loading in assessment of patients with renal disease. Am J Med 77: 873–9.
9. Bosch JP, Lew S, Glabman S, Lauer A, 1986: Renal hemodynamic changes in humans. Response to protein loading in normal and diseased kidneys. Am J Med 81: 809–15.
10. Hostetter TH, 1986: Human renal response to a meat meal. Am J Physiol 250: F613–F618.
11. Johannesen J, Lie M, Kiil F, 1977: Effect of glycine and glucagon on glomerular filtration and renal metabolic rates. Am J Physiol 233: F61–F66.
12. Lee KE, Summerill RA, 1982: Glomerular filtration rate following administration of individual aminoacids in conscious dogs. Quart J Exptl Physiol 67: 459–65.
13. Graf H, Stummvoll HK, Luger A, Prager R, 1983: Effects of aminoacid infusion on glomerular filtration rate. New Engl J Med 308: 159–60.
14. Meyer TW, Ichikawa I, Zatz R, Brenner BM, 1983: The renal hemodynamic response to aminoacid infusion in the rat. Trans Ass Am Phys 96: 76–83.
15. Palmore WP, 1983: Glucagon and alanine-induced increases of the canine renal glomerular filtration rate. Quart J Exptl Physiol 68: 319–27.
16. ter Wee PM, Geerlings W, Rosman JB, Sluiter WJ, van der Geest S, Donker Ab JM, 1985: Testing renal reserve filtration capacity with an aminoacid solution. Nephron 41: 193–9.

20

17. ter Wee PM, Rosman JB, van der Geest S, Sluiter WJ, Donker Ab JM, 1986: Renal hemodynamics during separate and combined infusion of aminoacids and dopamine. Kidney Int 29: 870–4.
18. Castellino P, Coda B, DeFronzo RA, 1986: Effect of aminoacid infusion on renal hemodynamics in humans. Am J Physiol 251: F132–F140.
19. Amiel C, Friedlander G, Blanchet F, Nitenberg A, Assan R, 1987: Aminoacid induced hyperfiltration in man is a glucagon mediated effect. Kidney Int 31: 418.
20. Hirschberg R, Kopple JD, 1987: Role of growth hormone in the aminoacid-induced acute rise in renal function in man. Kidney Int 32: 382–7.
21. Hirschberg R, Zipser RD, Slomowitz LA, Kopple JD, 1988: Glucagon and prostaglandins are mediators of aminoacid-induced rise in renal hemodynamics. Kidney Int 33: 1147–55.
22. Ruilope LM, Rodicio J, Robles RG et al., 1987: Influence of low sodium diet on the renal response to aminoacid infusions in humans. Kidney Int 31: 992–9.
23. Friedlander G, Blanchet-Benqué F, Nitenberg A, Laborie C, Assan R, Amiel C, in press: Glucagon secretion in essential for aminoacid-induced hyperfiltration in man. Nephrology transplantation and dialysis.
24. Premen AJ, 1989: Nature of the renal hemodynamic action of aminoacids in dogs. Am J Physiol 256: F516–F523.
25. Levy M, Starr NL, 1972: The mechanisms of glucagon-induced natriuresis in dogs. Kidney Int 2: 76–84.
26. Levy M, 1975: Further observations on the response of the glomerular filtration rate to glucagon: Comparison with secretion. Can J Physiol Pharmacol 53: 81–5.
27. Parving HH, Noer I, Kehlet H, Mogensen CE, Svendsen PAa, Heding L, 1977: The effect of short-term glucagon infusion on kidney function in normal man. Diabetologia 13: 323–5.
28. Bailly C, Roinel N, Amiel C, 1984: PTH-like glucagon stimulation of Ca and Mg reabsorption in Henle's loop of the rat. Am J Physiol 246: F205–F212.
29. Friedlander G, Blanchet-Benqué F, Bailly C, Assan R, Amiel C, 1985: Effets tubulaires rénaux du glucagon chez l'homme. Médecine/Sciences 1: 100–3.
30. Premen AJ, 1985: Importance of the liver during glucagon-mediated increases in canine renal hemodynamics. Am J Physiol 249: F319–F322.
31. Premen AJ, Hall JE, Smith MJ, 1985: Postprandial regulation of renal hemodynamics: Role of pancreatic glucagon. Am J Physiol 248: F656–F662.
32. Seney FD, Wright FS, 1985: Dietary protein suppresses feedback control of glomerular filtration in rats. J Clin Invest 75: 558–68.
33. Woods, LL, Leland Mizelle H, Montani JP, Hall JE, 1986: Mechanisms controlling renal hemodynamics and electrolyte excretion during aminoacids. Am J Physiol 251: F303–F312.
34. Seney FD, Persson AEG, Wright FS, 1987: Modification of tubuloglomerular feedback signal by dietary protein. Am J Physiol 252: F83–F90.
35. Bouby N, Trinh-Trang-Tan MM, Laouari D et al., 1988: Role of the urinary concentrating process in the renal effects of high protein intake. Kidney Int 34: 4–12.
36. Corman B, Chami-Khazraji S, Schaeverbeke J, Michel JB, 1988: Effect of feeding on glomerular filtration rate and proteinuria in conscious aging rats. Am J Physiol 255: F250–F256.

37. Paller MS, Hostetter TH, 1986: Dietary protein increases plasma renin and reduces pressor reactivity to angiotensin II. Am J Physiol 251: F34–F39.
38. Knopf RF, Conn JW, Fajans SS, Floyd JC, Guntsche EM, Rull JA, 1965: Plasma growth hormone response to intravenous administration of aminoacids. Am J Endocrinol 25: 1140–4.
39. Corvilain J, Abramow M, 1962: Some effects of human growth hormone on renal hemodynamics and on tubular phosphate transport in man. J Clin Invest 41: 1230–5.
40. Christiansen JS, Gammelgaard Orskov H, Anderson AR, Telmo S, Parving HH, 1981: Kidney function and size in normal subjects before and during growth hormone administration for one week. Eur J Clin Invest 11: 487–90.
41. Ikkos D, Ljunggren R, Luft R, 1957: Glomerular filtration rate and renal plasma flow in acromegaly. Acta Endocrinol 21: 226–36.
42. Kleinman KS, Glassock RJ, 1986: Glomerular filtration rate fails to increase following protein ingestion in hypothalamo-hypophyseal-deficient adults. Am J Nephrol 6: 169–74.
43. Hirschberg R, Rabb H, Bergamo R, Kopple JD, 1989: The delayed effect of growth hormone on renal function in humans. Kidney Int 35: 865–70.
44. Hirschberg R, Kopple JD, 1989: Evidence that insulin-like growth factor I increases renal plasma flow and glomerular filtration rate in fasted rats. J Clin Invest 83: 326–30.
45. Ohneda A, Parada E, Eisentraut AM, Unger RH, 1968. Characterization of response of circulating glucagon to intraduodenal and intravenous administration of aminoacids. J Clin Invest 47: 2305–22.
46. Unger RH, Aguilar-Parada E, Muller WA, Eisentraut AM, 1970: Studies of pancreatic alpha cell function in normal and diabetic subjects. J Clin Invest 49: 837–48.
47. Müller WA, Faloona GR, Unger RH, 1971: The effect of alanine on glucagon secretion. J Clin Invest 50: 2215–18.
48. Rocha DM, Faloona GR, Unger RH, 1972: Glucagon-stimulating activity of 20 aminoacids in dogs. J Clin Invest 51: 2346–51.
49. Unger RH, Orci L, 1976: Physiology and pathophysiology of glucagon. Physiol Rev 50: 778–826.
50. Bergström J, Ahlberg M, Alvestrand A, 1985: Influence of protein intake on renal hemodynamics and plasma hormone concentrations in normal subjects. Acta Med Scand 217: 189–96.
51. Assan R, Marre M, Gormley M, 1983: The aminoacid-induced secretion of glucagon. In Glucagon II. PJ Lefebvre (ed). Springer-Verlag, Berlin, pp. 19–41.
52. Okamura T, Miyazaki M, Toda N, 1986: Responses of isolated dog blood vessels to glucagon. Eur J Pharmacol 125: 395–401.
53. Premen AJ, 1987: Splanchnic and renal hemodynamic responses to intraportal infusion of glucagon. Am J Physiol 253: F1105–F1112.
54. Alvestrand A, Bergström J, 1984: Glomerular hyperfiltration after protein ingestion, during glucagon infusion, and in insulin-dependent diabetes is induced by a liver hormone: Deficient production of this hormone in hepatic failure causes hepatorenal syndrome. Lancet, 28 Jan, 195–7.
55. Premen AJ, 1986: Protein-mediated elevations in renal hemodynamics: Existence of a hepato-renal axis? Medical Hypotheses 19: 295–309.
56. Uranga J, Fuenzalida R, Rapoport AL, del Castillo E, 1979: Effect of glucagon and

glomerulopressin on the renal function of the dog. Horm Metab Res 11: 275–9.

57. Hirschberg R, von Herrath D, Pauls A, Schaefer K, 1984: No rise in glomerular filtration rate after protein load in severe liver disease. Lancet 3 Nov, 1047–8.

58. Levy M, 1978: Inability of glucagon to increase glomerular filtration rate in dogs with experimental cirrhosis and ascites. Can J Physiol Pharmacol 56: 511–14.

59. Woods LL, Leland Mizelle H, Hall JE, 1987: Role of the liver in renal hemodynamic response to aminoacid infusion. Am J Physiol 252: F981–F985.

60. Uranga J, 1971: Some characteristics of hepatic glomerular pressure substance. Am J Physiol 220: 1617–20.

61. Uranga J, Fuenzalida R, 1975: Effect of glomerulopressin and a rabbit glomerulopressin-like substance in the rat. Horm Metab Res 7: 180–4.

62. del Castillo E, Fuenzalida R, Uranga J, 1977: Increased glomerular filtration rate and glomerulopressin activity in diabetic dogs. Horm Metab Res 9: 46–53.

63. del Castillo E, Rapoport AL, Bonetto R, Uranga J, 1981: Glomerulopressin in dogs' mesenteric blood flow and protaglandins. Horm Metab Res 13: 126–7.

64. Zimmerman L, Alvestrand A, Bergström J, 1989: Elevated concentration of 5-hydroxytryptamine in ultrafiltrate of human liver vein plasma after infusion of aminoacids. Acta Physiol Scan (in press).

65. Levine MM, Kirschenbaum MA, Chaudhari A, Wong MW, Bricker NS, 1986: Effect of protein on glomerular filtration rate and prostanoid synthesis in normal and uremic rats. Am J Physiol 251: F635–F641.

66. Vanrenterghem YFCh, Verberckmoes RKA, Roels LM, Michielsen PJ, 1988: Role of prostaglandins in protein-induced glomerular hyperfiltration in normal humans. Am J Physiol 254: F463–F469.

67. Benigni A, Zoja C, Remuzzi A, Orisio S, Piccinelli A, Remuzzi G, 1986: Role of renal prostaglandins in normal and nephrotic rats with diet-induced hyperfiltration. J Lab Clin Med 108: 230–40.

68. Stahl RA, Kudelka S, Helmchen U, 1987: High protein intake stimulates glomerular prostaglandin formation in remnant kidney. Am J Physiol 252: F1083–F1094.

69. Knauss T, Abboud HE, 1986: Effect of serotonin on prostaglandins synthesis in rat cultured mesangial cells. Am J Physiol 251: F844–F850.

70. Blackshear JL, Orlandi C, Hollenberg NK, 1986: Serotonin and the renal blood supply: Role of prostaglandins and the 5HT-2 receptor. Kidney Int 30: 304–10.

71. Castellino P, Giordano C, Perna A, DeFronzo RA, 1988: Effects of plasma aminoacid and hormone levels on renal hemodynamics in humans. Am J Physiol 255: F444–F449.

72. Rodriguez-Iturbe B, Herrera J, Garcia R, 1985: Response to acute protein load in kidney donors and in apparently normal postacute glomerulonephritis patients: Evidence for glomerular hyperfiltration. Lancet 31 Aug, 461–5.

73. Dhaene M, Sabot JP, Philippart Y, Doutrelepont JM, Vanherweghem JL, Toussaint C, 1986: Renal functional reserve of transplanted kidney. Nephron 44: 157–8.

74. Tapson JS, Mansy H, Marshall SM, Tisdall SR, Wilkinson R, 1986: Renal functional reserve in kidney donors. Quart J Med 60: 725–32.

75. Rugiu C, Oldrizzi L, Maschio G, 1987: Effects of an oral protein load on glomerular filtration rate in patients with solitary kidneys. Kidney Int 32, suppl. 22: S29–S31.

76. Mogensen CE, 1986: Early glomerular hyperfiltration in insulin-dependent diabetics and late nephropathy. Scand J Clin Lab Invest 46: 201–6.

77. O'Donnell MP, Kasiske BL, Keane WF, 1988: Glomerular hemodynamic and structural alterations in experimental diabetes mellitus. FASEB 2: 2339–47.
78. Wiseman MJ, Saunders AJ, Keen H, Viberti GC, 1985: Effect of blood glucose control on increased glomerular filtration rate and kidney size in insulin-dependent diabetes. New Eng J Med 312: 617–21.
79. Wiseman MJ, Mangili R, Alberetto M, Keen H, Viberti G, 1987: Glomerular response mechanisms to glycemic changes in insulin-dependent diabetics. Kidney Int 31: 1012–18.
80. Woods LL, Leland Mizelle H, Hall JE, 1987: Control of renal hemodynamics in hyperglycemia: Possible role of tubuloglomerular feedback. Am J Physiol 252: F65–F73.
81. Parving HH, Christiansen JS, Noer I, Tronier B, Mogensen CE, 1980: The effect of glucagon infusion on kidney function in short-term insulin-dependent juvenile diabetics. Diabetologia 19: 350–4.
82. Wiseman MJ, Redmond S, House F, Keen H, Viberti GC, 1985: The glomerular hyperfiltration of diabetes is not associated with elevated plasma levels of glucagon and growth hormone. Diabetologia 28: 718–21.
83. Schambelan M, Blake S, Sraër J, Bens M, Nivez MP, Wahbe F, 1985: Increased prostaglandin production by glomeruli isolated from rats with streptozotocin-induced diabetes mellitus. J Clin Invest 75: 404–12.
84. Craven PA, Caines MA, DeRubertis FR, 1987: Sequential alterations in glomerular prostaglandin and thromboxane synthesis in diabetic rats: Relationship to the hyperfiltration of early diabetes. Metabolism 36: 95–103.
85. Ortola FV, Ballermann BJ, Anderson S, Mendez RE, Brenner BM, 1985: Elevated plasma atrial natriuretic peptide levels in diabetic rats. Potential mediator of hyperfiltration. J Clin Invest 80: 670–4.
86. Kupin WL, Cortes P, Dumler F, Feldkamp CS, Kilates MC, Levin NW, 1987: Effect on renal function of change from high to moderate protein intake in type I diabetic patients. Diabetes 36: 73–9.
87. Hirose K, Tsuchida H, Osterby R, Gundersen HJG, 1980: A strong correlation between glomerular filtration rate and filtration surface in diabetic kidney hyperfunction. Lab Invest 43: 434–7.
88. Ellis EN, Steffes MW, Goetz FC, Sutherland DER, Mauer SM, 1986: Glomerular filtration surface in type I diabetes mellitus. Kidney Int 29: 889–94.
89. Yoshida Y, Fogo A, Shiraga H, Glick AD, Ichikawa I, 1988: Serial micropuncture analysis of single nephron function in subtotal renal ablation. Kidney Int 33: 855–67.
90. Bertani T, Poggi A, Pozzoni R, Delaini F, Sacchi G, Thoua Y, Mecca G, Remuzzi G, Donati MB, 1982: Adriamycin-induced nephrotic syndrome in rats. Lab Invest 46: 16.
91. Grond J, Weening JJ, Elema JD, 1984: Glomerular sclerosis in nephrotic rats. Comparison of the long-term effects of adriamycin and aminonucleoside. Lab Invest 51: 277.
92. Nath KA, Kren SM, Hostetter TH, 1986: Dietary protein restriction in established renal injury in the rat: selective role of glomerular capillary pressure in progressive glomerular dysfunction. J Clin Invest 78: 1199–1205.
93. Molina E, Herrera J, Rodriguez-Iturbe B, 1988: The renal functional reserve in health and renal disease in school age children. Kidney Int 34, 809–16.

Angiotensin I – Converting enzyme inhibition in models of progressive glomerulosclerosis

JAN J. WEENING, PIETER J. WESTENEND & JORIS GROND

Studies in experimental models have revealed that several pathogenetic mechanisms may lead to focal glomerulosclerosis (FGS) associated with proteinuria and loss of renal function. These pathogenetic mechanisms can be separated into primary events (Figure 1) in which the glomerular capillary tuft is exposed to harmful stimuli such as hypertension with mechanical stress, toxic compounds, and high levels of circulatory lipids, glucose or other metabolic factors [1–3]. A sequence of secondary events includes endothelial cell damage and thrombosis, leukocyte influx, endothelial and mesangial cell proliferation, excessive lipid accumulation and matrix production, glomerular hypertrophy with volume expansion and epithelial cell damage with detachment and hyalinosis [4] (see Figure 1).

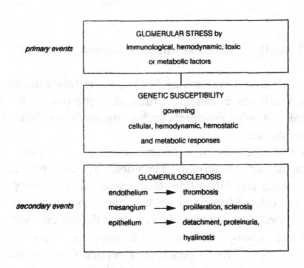

Figure 1. Adapted from Reference [5].

M. E. De Broe and G. A. Verpooten (eds.): Prevention in Nephrology, 25–38.
© 1991 *Kluwer Academic Publishers. Printed in the Netherlands.*

Genetic susceptibility has been shown to determine the extent to which afferent resistance protects the glomerular capillary tuft from transmitting the high systemic blood pressure in models of systemic hypertension and partial renal ablation [6, 7, 8]. It also determines the extent of epithelial cell damage and proteinuria after exposure to toxic components such as puromycin aminonucleoside [9].

Pharmaceutical or dietary intervention in FGS should be aimed at prevention by correction of the primary events or at inhibition of one or more of the secondary responses, e.g., when hemodynamic derangement with glomerular hypertension is of primary importance, as has been demonstrated in a number of experimental models [1, 4, 10–14], therapy should reduce the transcapillary pressure difference. At the level of secondary events, anti-coagulatory and lipid-lowering regimens may contribute to restriction of glomerular damage [15–18].

Angiotensin I-converting enzyme inhibition (ACEi) has been shown to be one of the most effective therapeutic maneuvers in the prevention of some experimental forms of FGS, characterized by elevated intraglomerular hydraulic pressure [5, 19–29]. As will be discussed in this chapter, ACEi exerts this beneficial effect primarily through a reduction in systemic and glomerular capillary pressure due to efferent vasodilation. By inhibiting the growth stimulating effect of angiotensin II (A II) ACEi may, in addition, reduce cell proliferation, one of the detrimental secondary events in FGS [30–32].

A II, ACEi and the glomerular microcirculation

Glomerular filtration is determined by the plasma flow rate, the transcapillary pressure difference and the structural properties of the glomerular capillary wall (GCW) components such as hydraulic conductivity and total filtration surface area.

Afferent and efferent arteriolar resistances play a crucial role in the maintenance of optimal filtration conditions by regulating the access of systemic pressure and blood flow to the vulnerable capillary network. In this respect, local production, activation, and binding of vasoactive substances by arteriolar endothelial and smooth muscle and glomerular endothelial and mesangial cells provide an important regulatory network of checks and balances. The vasoconstrictor peptide A II operates both in an endocrine, paracrine, as well as autocrine fashion [33]. A II receptors have been identified on mesangial cells and on the efferent arteriole. Systemic infusion of A II induces an increase of renovascular resistance, a reduction of RPF, an increase in transcapillary pressure and preservation or little change of GFR, possibly mediated by mesangial cell contraction [34]. Contraction of mesangial cells may lead to a reduction of the surface area available for ultrafiltration. In addition, systemic A II infusion into rats has been shown to cause mesangial accumulation of circulating macromolecules, an effect which could be prevented by competitive A II blockade with Saralasin [35].

A II blockade by Saralasin and ACEi by Captopril and Enalapril substantially reduces renovascular resistance, primarily through efferent arteriolar vasodilation, associated with a reduction in glomerular transcapillary pressure with preservation of GFR. Reduced intracapillary pressure probably underlies the beneficial effect of long term ACEi on the development of FGS in experimental models in the rat associated with disproportionate afferent dilation and glomerular capillary hypertension such as the remnant kidney, spontaneous hypertension, uninephrectomized normo- and hypertensive rats, high dietary protein feeding, streptozotocin-induced diabetes mellitus and puromycin aminonucleoside treated rats (see below). These experimental studies have also indicated that ACEi with preservation of GFR in conditions of established GCW damage with massive proteinuria, has neither a beneficial effect on protein loss nor on progressive deterioration of glomerular function and structure [36, 37]. At this stage, afferent vasoconstriction, e.g. by dietary protein restriction or by a combination of ACEi and salt restriction, may be the only way to limit glomerular disease.

We studied the effect of ACEi by Captopril on renal functional and structural parameters in three models of FGS. In the first study (*Renal Ablation*) [21], Captopril was given to groups of uninephrectomized normotensive male Wistar rats either from early on, that is starting ACEi immediately after uninephrectomy, or after a therapy-free interval of 7 months at which time the animals had developed overt proteinuria and FGS. The second model was *Adriamycin Nephrosis* in female normotensive Wistar rats [36]. The effect of ACEi was compared with that of dietary protein restriction. In the third study (*Fawn Hooded*) [27], spontaneously hypertensive Fawn Hooded rats (FH), which are particularly susceptible to develop proteinuria and progressive glomerulosclerosis, were treated with Captopril and studied for their response in systemic blood pressure, urinary protein loss, incidence of FGS lesions, glomerular volume expansion, and renal function.

28

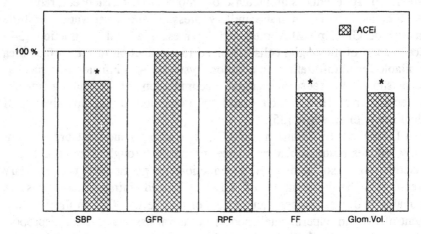

Figure 2. Effects of early treatment with ACEi on SBP, GFR, RPF, FF and glomerular volume in uninephrectomized Wistar rats. Control values set at 100%, *P < 0.05. Student's T-test (adapted from Reference [21]).

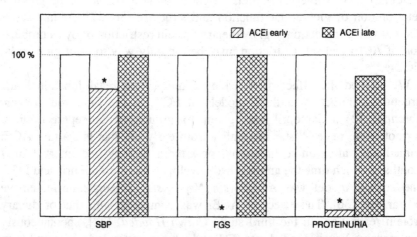

Figure 3. Effects of ACEi early or late treatment on SBP, FGS and proteinuria in uninephrectomized Wistar rats. Control values set at 100%, *P < 0.05 anova (adapted from Reference [21]).

Renal ablation

ACEi, when started early from the moment of uninephrectomy, lowered systemic blood pressure and prevented the development of proteinuria and FGS (Figure 2). Renal functional studies revealed a significant reduction of FF by ACEi, with preservation of GFR, indicative of a decrease in glomerular transcapillary pressure difference. Glomerular volume expansion with structural hypertrophy in the untreated uninephrectomized animals was prevented by ACEi (Figure 2). These beneficial effects of ACEi, i.e. prevention of FGS by early treatment, were not found when Captopril was started later at the time when glomerular damage was established. In these rats urinary protein loss further increased from a median value of 265 mg per 24 hours to 355 (control group 223 to 484 mg per 24 hours) notwithstanding ACEi (Figure 3). The incidence of FGS lesions was approximately 40% in the Captopril as well as in the control group. The lack of effect of ACEi on the progression of FGS under these conditions was associated with a therapy resistance of the animals' systemic blood pressure (Figure 3) in contrast to the early treatment group, possibly due to structural changes in the efferent vessel wall or a loss of tubulo-glomerular feedback inhibition.

This study indicates that after unilateral nephrectomy and concomitant afferent vasodilation, early ACEi normalizes glomerular transcapillary pressure by efferent vasodilation, as evidenced by the reduction in FF. This, in turn, may prevent glomerular volume expansion, endothelial and epithelial cell injury, and mesangial overloading. In this respect, the response in the normotensive unilateral nephrectomy model is very similar to that in the remnant kidney model, in which five-sixth of the total kidney mass is ablated by unilateral nephrectomy and infarction of two-third part of the remaining kidney. Anderson *et al.* studied the effect of early ACEi by Enalapril in this more aggressive model of renal ablation associated with systemic hypertension [19]. Treatment with ACEi prevented systemic hypertension and nearly normalized the intraglomerular pressure gradient associated with a significant limitation of proteinuria and glomerular injury. In a second study in the same experimental model, these workers showed that the beneficial effects of ACEi are directly related to the normalization of intraglomerular pressure rather than to that of the systemic blood pressure. Treatment with a combination of reserpine, hydralazine and hydrochloro-thiazide resulted in a similar reduction of systemic hypertension as accomplished by ACEi. However, intraglomerular pressure was still elevated and the triple drug regimen failed to prevent the development of FGS. In contrast to our finding that ACEi did not limit the progression of FGS when given at a later stage, Meyer *et al.* [24] reported a reduction of intraglomerular pressure with stabilization of proteinuria and glomerular injury by starting treatment with ACEi or dietary protein restriction in the remnant kidney model after a therapy-free interval of 8 weeks when the animals had developed severe systemic hypertension, proteinuria and FGS. To further analyse the effects of ACEi on progressive glomerulosclerosis in established forms of glomerular injury, we studied ACEi in Adriamycin-induced nephrosis and compared the effects with those of dietary protein restriction [36].

Adriamycin nephrosis

After induction of Adriamycin Nephrosis by a single i.v. dose of Adriamycin (3 mg per kg body weight), animals were randomized over six experimental groups. One group was maintained on a 22% protein diet and one on an isocaloric 6% protein diet. Both groups were followed for approximately 80 days. Two other groups were started on a 22 and 6% protein diet, respectively. Halfway during the observation period, the rats were switched to the alternative diet. Two more groups were started on ACEi by Captopril, one for the full observation period, one for the first half only. Two control groups were included that received no Adriamycin and were maintained on a 22 or 6% protein diet, respectively. Renal function studies were performed in six separate groups on the same regimens. Whereas dietary protein restriction was found to reduce urinary protein loss (Figure 4), glomerular volume expansion and the incidence of FGS lesions considerably, ACEi had no effect on these parameters when compared to controls, even though ACEi was associated with a marked fall in systemic blood pressure (Figure 5). Renal function studies revealed that dietary protein restriction lowered GFR numerically and RPF significantly (concordant with other studies on dietary protein restriction), whereas ACEi had no effect on GFR or RPF (Figure 6).

From these data, we concluded that the effect of protein restriction might be partially hemodynamically mediated by afferent vasoconstriction resulting in a decrease in GFR and a reduction in protein flux across the Adriamycin-induced large pore defects in the glomerular capillary wall [36].

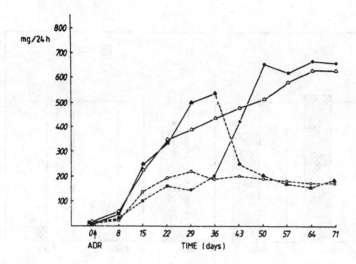

Figure 4. Mean urinary protein excretion of ADR-treated rats on an LP (- - -) or a NP (————) protein diet.

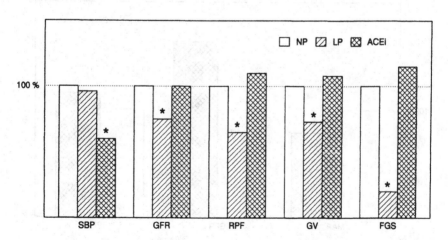

Figure 5. Effects of normal (NP) and low protein (LP) diet and ACEi on SPB, GFR, RPF, GV and FGS in adriamycin nephrosis. NP values set at 100%, *P < 0.05 anova (adapted from Reference [36]).

32

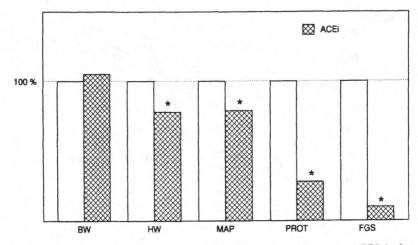

Figure 6. Effects of ACEi on body and heart weights, map, proteinuria and FGS in fawn-hooded rats at 12 months. Control values set at 100%, *P < 0.05. Student's T-test (adapted from Reference [27]).

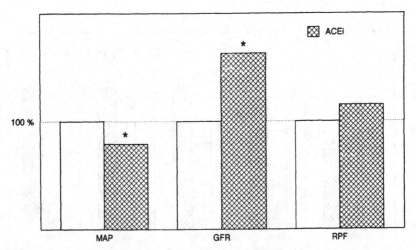

Figure 7. Effects of ACEi on map, GFR and RPF in fawn-hooded rats. Control values set at 100%, *P < 0.05. Student's T-test (adapted from Reference [27]).

Maintenance of GFR in this model, as seen under ACEi, allows the same amount of proteins to be filtered as under control conditions. The protein leak in itself may lead to further glomerular epithelial cell injury [38] and tubular cast formation, ultimately contributing to progressive glomerulosclerosis. These findings are concordant with those of Scholey et al. [37] who performed micropuncture studies in Adriamycin nephrotic rats treated with ACEi. They found no effect of ACEi on proteinuria nor on FGS notwithstanding a reduction in systemic and intraglomerular pressure. Similarly, no effect of ACEi was found on the acute and chronic course of puromycin aminonucleoside nephrosis induced by repetitive administration of puromycin [26, 39]. This suggests, that under these circumstances of severe capillary wall damage with large pore defects, similar to established damage in the ablation model, ACEi may be beneficial only when combined with a dietary salt restriction as to lower GFR as well as transcapillary pressure. Indication for the usefulness of this kind of intervention is provided by the clinical studies of Heeg et al. [40].

Fawn Hooded

The Fawn Hooded rat develops systemic hypertension and FGS relatively early in life and suffers from progressive loss of renal function leading to end-stage renal failure [41, 42]. In its susceptibility to develop FGS, the FH rat resembles the Dahl S rat and contrasts with the SHR and Milan Hypertensive stain which are relatively resistant to the development of FGS, due to a high afferent resistance [7, 8]. The effects of ACEi by Captopril were studied in intact FH, treated from the age of 5 months. Renal function parameters measured after one month of ACEi revealed a markedly higher GFR in the Captopril treated rats as compared to controls, notwithstanding a significant reduction in systemic blood pressure (Figure 7). RPF was not significantly increased. Notwithstanding the higher GFR, possibly due to effects on Kf, at sacrifice at 12 months of age, the Captopril treated rats were found to have significantly lower values for heart weight, mean arterial blood pressure, incidence of FGS, and urinary protein loss. No differences were found for glomerular volume expansion [27] (Figure 7).

Other studies have shown that early treatment by ACEi prevents or limits FGS in uninephrectomized SHR rats [22] and in experimental diabetes mellitus [28]. Triple drug therapy was also effective in the SHR model but not in the experimental diabetes. Recently, Anderson et al. [25] studied

ACEi by Captopril in Munich-Wistar rats which developed FGS after a long disease-free interval following acute puromycin aminonucleoside nephrosis. During the disease-free interval, glomerular intracapillary pressure was found to be elevated [25]. ACEi normalized the intra-glomerular hypertension and prevented the development of proteinuria and FGS.

ACEi in diagnosis

Apart from its usefulness in the treatment of chronic glomerular disease leading to FGS, ACEi may also be helpful in recognizing FGS-suscep-tibility. As mentioned above, genetic differences exist in susceptibility to develop FGS after unilateral nephrectomy or administration of puromycin aminonucleoside. These differences may depend in part upon vascular reactivity governing the afferent-efferent balance of the glomerular circula-tion. A decrease in efferent resistance in the nephrons remaining after unilateral nephrectomy, may protect the capillary tuft from an increase in transcapillary pressure due to concomitant afferent vasodilation. Rats that do not adequately dilate the efferent arteriole in the case of compensatory hyperfiltration, will expose the glomerular capillaries to higher pressure, associated with an increase in FF, and will ultimately develop FGS. Most rats, but not all, seem to have difficulties in responding to loss of renal mass with adequate efferent vasodilation. We studied the acute responses in GFR, RPF, FF and renovascular resistance (RVR) after a bolus injection of Captopril in two normotensive Wistar rat strains, one of which (Wistar Zeist) is susceptible to develop FGS after unilateral nephrectomy and one of which (Wistar Kyoto) is resistant. Both intact and uninephrectomized (UN) rats were studied. FF and RVR were found to be higher in intact and UN Wistar Zeist rats and after an i.v. injection of Captopril at 10 mg per kg, FF was found to be reduced by approximately 50% in intact and UN FGS susceptible Wistar Zeist rats and by only 20% in UN Wistar Kyoto rats (Figure 8), RVR decreased with 25% in intact and UN Wistar Zeist, but not in Wistar Kyoto (Figure 9). These results indicate efferent vasoconstriction in the FGS-susceptible strain which can be influenced by ACEi. In Wistar Kyoto rats, efferent vasodilation seems to be near maximal and shows little additional effect after ACEi.

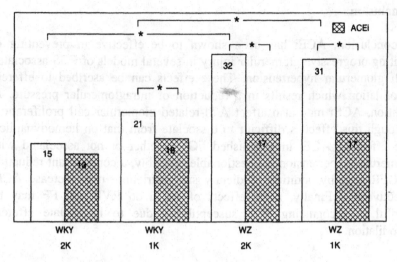

Figure 8. Effects of acute ACEi on filtration fraction in intact or uninephrectomized WKY and WZ rats. Values are means for filtration fraction, *P < 0.05 anova.

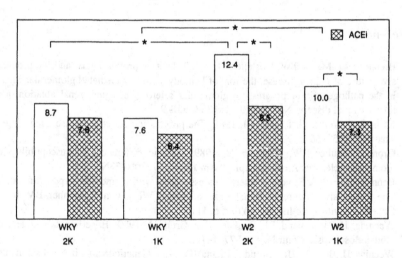

Figure 9. Effects of acute ACEi on renovascular resistance in intact or uninephrectomized WKY and WZ rats. Values are means for renovascular resistance, *P < 0.05 anova.

Conclusion

In conclusion, ACEi has been shown to be effective in preventing or limiting progressive glomerular injury in several models of FGS associated with glomerular hypertension. These effects can be ascribed to efferent vasodilation which results in a reduction of intraglomerular pressure. In addition, ACEi may also affect A II-related glomerular cell proliferation, although this effect is difficult to dissociate from that on hemodynamics. The effect of ACEi in established FGS whether or not associated with glomerular hypertension is questionable. Possibly, a concomitant reduction in GFR, e.g. by addition of dietary salt restriction, may increase ACEi effectiveness. Finally, acute effects of ACEi on RVR and FF may be helpful in recognizing FGS susceptibility due to inadequate efferent vasodilation.

Acknowledgements

This work was supported by grants from the Dutch Kidney Foundation and the Prevention Fund

References

1. Brenner BM, Meyer TW, Hostetter TH, 1982: Dietary protein intake and the progressive nature of kidney disease: the role of hemodynamically mediated glomerular injury in the pathogenesis of progressive glomerular sclerosis in aging, renal ablation, and intrinsic renal disease. New Engl J Med 307: 651–9.
2. Klahr S, Schreiner G, Ichikawa I, 1988: The progression of renal disease. New Engl J Med 318: 1657–66.
3. Grond J, Muller EW, Weening JJ, 1989: Genetic differences in susceptibility to glomerular sclerosis. A role for lipids? Am J Med, 87: 30N–33N.
4. Rennke HG, 1986: Structural alterations associated with glomerular hyperfiltration, in The Progressive Nature of Renal Disease, Mitch WE, Stein J, Brenner BM (eds). Churchill Livingstone Inc, New York, p. 111.
5. Weening JJ, Westenend PJ, Beukers JJB, Grond J, 1989: Experimental models of glomerulosclerosis. Contr Nephrol 77: 1–12.
6. Weening JJ, Beukers JJB, Grond J, Elema JD, 1986: Genetic factors in focal segmental glomerulosclerosis. Kidney Int 29: 789–98.
7. Dworkin LD, Feiner HD, 1986: Glomerular injury in uninephrectomized spontaneously hypertensive rats. A consequence of glomerular capillary hypertension. J Clin Invest 77: 797–809.

8. Brandis A, Bianchi G, Reale E, Helmchen U, Kühn K, 1986: Age-dependent glomerulosclerosis and proteinuria occurring in rats of the Milan normotensive strain and not in rats of the Milan hypertensive strain. Lab Invest 55: 234–43.

9. Grond J, Muller EW, Goor H van, Weening JJ, Elema JD, 1988: Interstrain differences in puromycin animonucleoside nephrosis in rats. Kidney Int 33: 524–9.

10. Hostetter TH, Olson JL, Rennke HG, Venkatachalam MA, Brenner BM, 1981: Hyperfiltration in remnant nephrons: A potentially adverse response to renal ablation. Am J Physiol 241: F85–F93.

11. Olson JL, Hostetter TH, Rennke HG, Brenner BM, Venkatachalam MA, 1982: Altered glomerular permselectivity and progressive sclerosis following extreme ablation of renal mass. Kidney Int 22: 112–26.

12. Hostetter TH, Troy JL, Brenner BM, 1981: Glomerular hemodynamics in experimental diabetes mellitus. Kidney Int 19: 410–15.

13. Zatz R, Meyer TW, Rennke HG, Brenner BM, 1985: Predominance of hemodynamic rather than metabolic factors in the pathogenesis of diabetic glomerulopathy. Proc Natl Acad Sci USA 82: 5963–67.

14. Dworkin LD, Hostetter TH, Rennke HG, Brenner BM, 1984: Hemodynamic basis for glomerular injury in rats with desoxycortico-sterone-salt hypertension. J Clin Invest 73: 1448–61.

15. Purkerson ML, Joist JH, Greenberg JM, Kay D, Hoffsten PE, Klahr S, 1982: Inhibition by anticoagulant drugs of the progressive hypertension and uremia associated with renal infarction in rats. Thromb Res 26: 227–40.

16. Olson JL, 1984: Role of heparin as a protective agent following reduction of renal mass. Kidney Int 25: 376–82.

17. Zoja C, Benigni A, Livio M, 1989: Selective inhibition of platelet thromboxane generation with low-dose aspirin does protect rats with reduced renal mass from the development of progressive disease. Am J Pathol 134: 1027–38.

18. Kasiske BL, O'Donnell MP, Garvis WJ, Keane WF, 1988: Pharmacologic treatment of hyperlipidimia reduces glomerular injury in the rat 5/6 nephrectomy model of chronic renal failure. Circ Res 62: 367–74.

19. Anderson S, Meyer TW, Rennke HG, Brenner BM, 1985: Control of glomerular hypertension limits glomerular injury in rats with reduced renal mass. J Clin Invest 76: 612–19.

20. Anderson S, Rennke HG, Brenner BM, 1986: Therapeutic advantage of converting enzyme inhibitors in arresting progressive renal disease associated with systemic hypertension in the rat. J Clin Invest 77: 1993–2000.

21. Beukers JJB, Wal A van der, Hoedemaeker PJ, Weening JJ, 1987: Converting enzyme inhibition and progressive glomerulosclerosis in the rat. Kidney Int 32: 794–800.

22. Zatz R, Dunn BR, Meyer TW, Anderson S, Rennke HG, Brenner BM, 1986: Prevention of diabetic glomerulopathy by pharmacological amelioration of glomerular capillary hypertension. J Clin Invest 77: 1925–30.

23. Anderson S, Rennke HG, Garcia DL, Brenner BM, 1989: Short and long term effects of antihypertensive therapy in the diabetic rat. Kidney Int 36: 526–36.

24. Meyer TW, Anderson S, Rennke HG, Brenner BM, 1987: Reversing glomerular hypertension stabilizes established glomerular injury. Kidney Int 31: 752–9.

38

25. Anderson S, Diamond JR, Karnovsky MJ, Brenner BM, 1988: Mechanisms underlying transition from acute glomerular injury to late glomerular sclerosis in a rat model of nephrotic syndrome. J Clin Invest 82: 1757–68.
26. Herrera-Acosta J, Gabbai F, Tapia E, et al., 1986: Effect of captopril and hycrochlorathiazide on glomerular hemodynamics and histological damage in Goldblatt hypertension with partial renal ablation. J Hypertension 4: S275–9.
27. Weening JJ, Westenend PJ, Nooyen Y, Brummelen P van, 1990: Monotherapy with ketanserin (K) is ineffective in lowering proteinuria or preventing glomerulosclerosis (GS) in the Fawn-Hooded rat (FH) whereas Captopril (CAP) is. Kidney Int, in press.
28. Dworkin, LD, Grosser M, Feiner HD, Ullian M, Parker M, 1989: Renal vascular effects of antihypertensive therapy in uninephrectomized SHR. Kidney Int 35: 790–8.
29. Yoshida Y, Kawamura T, Ikoma M, Fogo A, Ichikawa I, 1989: Effects of antihypertensive drugs on glomerular morphology. Kidney Int 36: 626–35.
30. Takama T, Kitamura H, Fujiwara Y, 1988: Effect of angiotensin II on DNA-synthesis in cultured rat mesangial cells. Kidney Int 33: 245 (abstract).
31. Ardaillou R, Sraer J, Chansel D, 1987: The effects of angiotensin II on isolated glomeruli and cultured glomerular cells. Kidney Int 31: S74–80.
32. Powell JS, Clozei JP, Muller RKM, Kuhn H, Hefti F, Hosang M, Baumgartner HR, 1989: Inhibitors of angiotensin-converting enzyme prevent myointimal proliferation after vascular injury. Science 245: 186–8.
33. Ehlers MRW, Riordan JF, 1989: Angiotensin-converting enzyme: New concepts concerning its biological role. Biochemistry 28: 5311–18.
34. Dworkin LD, Ichikawa I, Brenner BM, 1983: Hormonal modulation of glomerular function. Am J Physiol 244: F95–104.
35. Keane WF, Raij L, 1985: Relationship among altered glomerular barrier permselectivity, angiotensin II, and mesangial uptake of macromolecules. Lab Invest 52: 599–604.
36. Beukers JJB, Hoedemaeker PJ, Weening JJ, 1988: A comparison of the effects of converting-enzyme inhibition and protein restriction in experimental nephrosis. Lab Invest 59: 631–40.
37. Scholey JW, Miller PL, Rennke HG, Meyer TW, 1989: Effect of converting enzyme inhibition on the course of adriamycin-induced nephropathy. Kidney Int 36: 816–22.
38. Weening JJ, Guldener C van, Daha MR, Klar N, Wal A van der, Prins FA, 1987: The pathophysiology of protein-overload proteinuria. Am J Pathol 129: 64–73.
39. Marinides GN, Groggel GC, Cohen AH, Cook T, Baranowsky RL, Westenfelder C, Border WA, 1987: Failure of angiotensin converting enzyme inhibition to affect the course of chronic puromycin aminonucleoside nephropathy. Am J Pathol 129: 394–401.
40. Heeg JE, Jong PE de, Hem GK van der, Zeeuw D de, 1989: Efficacy and variability of the antiproteinuric effect of ACE inhibition by lisinopril. Kidney Int 36: 272–9.
41. Kreisberg JI, Karnovsky MJ, 1978: Focal glomerular sclerosis in the Fawn-Hooded rat. Am J Pathol 92:
42. Kuijpers MHM, Gruys E, 1984: Spontaneous hypertension and hypertensive renal disease in the Fawn-Hooded rat. Br J Exp Pathol 65: 181–90.

Prevention of nephrotoxicity of beta-lactam antibiotics

BRUCE M. TUNE & CHIEH-YIN HSU

Background

The beta-lactam antibiotics in current use include the penicillins, the cephalosporins, and the penems. With one exception, the penicillins have no direct renal toxicity. Although the same was expected from other beta-lactams, at least two cephalosporins and the first penem, N-formimidoyl-thienamycin (or imipenem), are highly nephrotoxic, and several other cephalosporins are mildly-to-moderately toxic to the kidney.

Pharmacologic studies of newly developed antibiotics are done in healthy laboratory animals, while toxicologic screening and subsequent clinical trials do not generally test potential toxic interactions. Thus, although acute renal failure is relatively common during serious infections, the clinician may not be fully aware of the contribution of the antibiotics used in their treatment. Studies in this laboratory, using the rabbit, have involved the mechanisms of nephrotoxicity of the beta-lactams and the potentiation of this toxicity by risk factors such as aminoglycosides, renal ischemia, and endotoxemia. To establish the basis for extrapolating from the animal model to the clinical setting, the present discussion will briefly review data regarding toxicity in humans, in nonhuman primates, and in other laboratory animals.

The beta-lactams most nephrotoxic in the rabbit are cephaloridine, cephaloglycin, and imipenem (Table 1) [1–5]. Cephaloridine produced enough renal injury in otherwise uncomplicated cases to provide a body of data regarding its toxicity to humans. Cephaloglycin, it appears, was not even tested in monkeys, but proved to be extremely toxic to the rabbit and was released only for oral use. Thus, cephaloglycin failed to produce the blood levels necessary to test its clinical toxicity. Imipenem has toxicity in rabbits and monkeys comparable to that of cephaloridine; it is marketed in

M. E. De Broe and G. A. Verpooten (eds.): Prevention in Nephrology, 39–49.

Table 1. Nephrotoxicity of three beta-lactam antibiotics in several animal species

	Rat[a]	Rabbit[a]	Monkey[a]	Human[b]
Cephaloridine [1, 2]	1200	100	300	≥100
Cephaloglycin [3, 4]	700	60	-	-
Imipenem [5]	≥1250	100	180	-

[a] Single parenteral doses that produce acute tubular necrosis in one-half of the animals treated (mg/kg BW).
[b] Approximate daily dose with a significant risk of acute nephrotoxicity.

Table 2. Additive toxicity of aminoglycosides and cephalothin in the human kidney

	A[a]	C[a]	A+C
Klastersky et al.[b]	6%	2%	21%
Wade et al.[c]	7%	-	26%
EORTC Group[d]	2%	4%	12%

% of patients with decreased renal function, as defined below.
[a] Aminoglycoside (A) and cephalothin (C) combined either with methicillin or ticarcillin or with one another (A+C).
[b] Tobramycin; serum creatinine → > 2.0 [7].
[c] Gentamicin or tobramycin; serum creatinine ↑ by ≥ 0.4 [8].
[d] Gentamicin; serum creatinine 1.5 → 2.5 [9].

Table 3. Impact of multiple risk factors on antibiotic nephrotoxicity (rabbit)

	Aminoglycoside[a]	Endotoxemia[b]	
	Cr_s[c]	Cr_s[c]	$Cr_s > 1.1$
C	0.74 ± 0.05	1.08 ± 0.12	2/12
A	0.95 ± 0.07	0.83 ± 0.03	0/12
E	-	0.76 ± 0.07	0/12
C+A	7.30 ± 2.24	0.77 ± 0.04	0/12
C+E	-	2.72 ± 1.12	4/12
A+E	-	3.04 ± 1.24	4/12
C+A+E	-	4.17 ± 1.20	11/12

Cephalosporin (C), aminoglycoside (A), and endotoxemia (E).
Data presented as serum creatinine (Cr_s, mg/dl) or numbers of animals with above-normal serum creatinine ($Cr_s > 1.1$).
[a] Cefaclor (300 mg/kg), gentamicin (100 mg/kg)/da × 5 da [4].
[b] Cephaloglycin (60 mg/kg), neomycin (60 mg/kg), endotoxin (0.5 mg/kg) in single doses [10].
[c] Normal serum creatinine = 0.79 ± SEM 0.03 ($n = 24$).

combination with cilastatin, an inhibitor of its enzymatic breakdown in the kidney that also inhibits its nephrotoxicity [5].

The data in Table 1 show potentially severe nephrotoxicity of three clinically released beta-lactams, and suggest that the rabbit, more than the rat, provides a suitable model for the study of their toxic potential. Several cephalosporins in common use, such as cefaclor, cefazolin, cefamandole, and to some extent cephalothin, are mildly-to-moderately toxic to the rabbit [6], and their potential for producing renal damage is increased by several clinical risk factors. The best described state of potentiated toxicity in human use is the cephalosporin-aminoglycoside synergy (Table 2) [7–9]. The three prospective, controlled series summarized here showed a significant increase of renal functional impairment (shown as percent of patients with increased serum creatinine concentrations) from combined compared to separate use of cephalothin and an aminoglycoside. Work in the rabbit suggests an even greater risk with more toxic cephalosporins like cefaclor and cefazolin [4].

Studies of the cephalosporin-aminoglycoside interactions in humans have been challenged because broad-spectrum penicillins may have decreased cephalosporin or aminoglycoside toxicity in the control groups. Table 3 demonstrates the cephalosporin-aminoglycoside synergy in rabbits in the absence of this variable [4, 10]. On the left are shown serum creatinine concentrations in rabbits given 5 days of a cefaclor-gentamicin combination in doses that caused little or no tubular necrosis or elevation of creatinine when given alone [4]. In combination, these two drugs were nephrotoxic to every animal treated. On the right are the results of separate and combined administration of single, minimally toxic doses of cephaloglycin and neomycin too small to produce a toxic synergy by themselves, but strongly toxic in combination with a single dose of bacterial cell wall lipopolysaccharide [10].

The combination of all three insults produced abnormal of serum creatinine concentrations in more animals than did the combination of any two of them. Although endotoxic shock is commonly blamed for the acute renal failure of bacterial septicemia, the 15% lethal dose of lipopolysaccharide used in these studies caused no tubular necrosis or increase of creatinine in survivors at the 48 hour time of sacrifice, although it was strongly additive with the nephrotoxic antibiotics.

Mechanisms of toxicity

Histopathologically, beta-lactam-induced renal injury is a purely proximal tubular necrosis [1, 6]. Four proposed mechanisms of this cytotoxicity have recently been reviewed [6]. These mechanisms are not necessarily in confict with one another. (1) *Tubular transport*. Early studies in this laboratory with cephaloridine, later confirmed with other cephalosporins, established a consistent relationship between secretory transport, resulting in high cellular concentrations, and the nephrotoxicity of the beta-lactams. (2) *MFO activation*. In 1977, McMurtry and Mitchell suggested that cephaloridine was converted by a cytochrome P-450 mixed function oxidase (MFO) to a highly reactive intermediate responsible for its nephrotoxicity. (3) *Lipid peroxidation*. In 1983, Kuo and associates, following a series of studies that failed to support the MFO hypothesis, demonstrated cephaloridine-induced lipid peroxidative injury and provided evidence for a role of this process in producing tubular necrosis. However, the molecular structures of various nephrotoxic and nontoxic beta-lactams indicated that this mechanism was not likely to apply to antibiotics other than cephaloridine. (4) *Mitochondrial injury*. In 1978, we proposed a role of mitochondrial injury. Recent studies with cephaloridine [11], cephaloglycin [12], and imipenem [13] have provided evidence against a major component of lipid peroxidation in the toxicity of the latter two compounds, and provide evidence that the respiratory injury produced by all three beta-lactams is the result of an attack on mitochondrial anionic substrate transporters – analogous to the mechanism by which this class of antibiotics inactivates bacterial membrane-bound proteins.

The present discussion will consider the sequential roles of tubular transport and the attack on mitochondrial substrate transporters in beta-lactam nephrotoxicity.

Tubular transport

Like benzylpenicillin, many of the cephalosporins are secreted across the proximal tubule by the *p*-aminohippurate carrier on the antiluminal side of the tubule, thereby reaching intracellular concentrations orders of magnitude greater than in any other cell type. Evidence of the toxicologic importance of this transport is as follows [6]: the occurrence of beta-lactam injury only with those antibiotics that undergo tubular secretion; its restriction to the proximal tubule; a correlation of cortical antibiotic concentra-

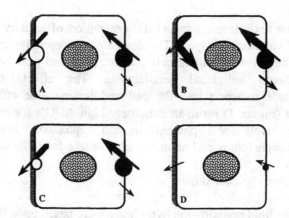

Figure 1. Movement of beta-lactam anbitiotics across the proximal renal tubular cell [6]. The antibiotics are actively transported into the tubular cell at the antiluminal (or blood) side; they then move down a concentration gradient into the tubular fluid, probably facilitated by a luminal transporter. (A) Normal movement, as seen with *p*- aminohippurate and as reflected in the renal uptake and secretion of cephalothin and cefaclor. (B) Severely restricted movement across the luminal membrane, as occurs with cephaloridine, resulting in extremely high and prolonged intracellular concentrations. (C) Partially restricted luminal-side movement, resulting in intermediate degrees of intracellular sequestration (e.g., cephaloglycin and cephalexin). (D) Minimal transport into the tubular cell (e.g., cef-tazidime).

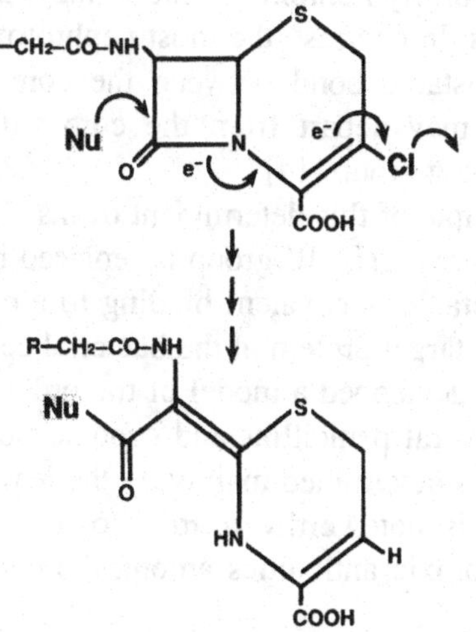

Figure 2. Departure of the chlorine atom (Cl) from cefaclor during attack by a nucleophile (Nu), such as an amino group. The resulting electron (e-) shifts destabilize the beta-lactam ring and facilitate acylation of the target protein.

tions with the toxic threshold; and the prevention of toxicity by different inhibitors of secretory transport. The degree of concentrative uptake, or the area under the curve of tubular cell concentration and time (AUC), varies greatly between individual beta-lactams. The effects of differing antiluminal-side transport into the cell and luminal-side efflux into the tubular fluid (Figure 1) result in extremely high AUC's for cephaloridine, intermediate levels for cephaloglycin and cephalexin, low levels for cefaclor and cephalothin, and no measurable uptake for ceftazidime [6].

Structure-activity relationships

The MFO and lipid peroxidation hypotheses were based upon the properties of specific sidegroup substituents not found on nephrotoxic beta-lactams other than cephaloridine [6]. A more comprehensive understanding of the molecular basis of injury required analysis of the structural properties common to all of the nephrotoxic beta-lactams. Examination of the side-group substituents on the toxic and nontoxic cephalosporins does not show common or even similar side-groups in the nephrotoxic ones [6]. However, one generalization could be taken from their structures: there is no nephrotoxic cephalosporin with an $R' = $ hydrogen in the $-CH2-R'$ sidegroup on the 3-carbon position of the cephalosporin ring. The penicillins, which are uniformly nontoxic to the kidney, also have a hydrogen at the equivalent locus. In contrast, the most nephrotoxic cephalosporins have a comparatively unstable bond between the core compound and the R' substituent, which may depart from the core structure and is therefore designated as a leaving group [14].

An extreme example of this determinant of instability is cefaclor (Figure 2), in which the entire $-CH2-R'$ group is replaced by $-Cl$, the departure of which facilitates cefaclor's covalent binding to a nucleophile, typically an amino group on the target protein in the bacterial cell membrane. Indelicato and associates [14] developed a model of the order of reactivity, or acylating potential, of several penicillins and cephalosporins. A 25- to 100-fold range of reactivity is determined mainly by the leaving properties of the R' side-groups. What is noteworthy from a toxicologic perspective, is that there are no nephrotoxic antibiotics among the comparatively stable beta-lactams.

Without exception, therefore, the nephrotoxic cephalosporins share two important properties, one or both of which are lacking in the nontoxic beta-lactams. First, in the kidney they undergo secretory uptake, reaching tubular cell concentrations up to thousands of times greater than in any other cell. Second, they have comparatively high reactivity or acylating potentials compared to other beta-lactams. As a result of their disproportionate intracellular sequestration and acylating activity, the nephrotoxic beta-lactams, such as cephaloglycin, bind covalently to membrane-bound proteins within the proximal tubular cell well out of proportion to the minimally toxic or nontoxic beta-lactams, such as cephalothin and benzyl-penicillin [6].

Mitochondrial toxicity

Several lines of evidence suggested that the toxic cephalosporins and imipenem produce tubular necrosis by causing mitochondrial respiratory toxicity [6]. Mitochondrial respiration is reduced *in situ* only by the nephrotoxic beta-lactams. Respiratory toxicity develops within one-half hour of administration of a single dose; is associated with cortical ATP depletion by 1-1/2 hours; and precedes ultrastructural damage by 5–10 hours. Finally, the resulting lesion resembles ischemic injury ultrastructurally. Three observations suggested an effect of the nephrotoxic beta-lactams on the transporters that carry anionic substrates into the mitochondrial inner matrix [6]. The first was their natural ability to acylate and inactivate membrane-bound proteins. Second, their greater toxicity to respiration with succinate, which donates electrons to the mid-region of the cytochrome chain, than to respiration with glutamate and malate, which donate electrons proximal to that locus, indicates an action outside the electron transport chain. Finally, respiratory toxicity can be reversed early in the process by increasing concentrations of substrate, reflected as an increased k_m for succinate with an unaffected V_{max} in studies of *in vitro* toxicity [15].

This early competitive inhibition suggests that, while all beta-lactams may fit the mitochondrial carriers for anionic substrate transport, *in vivo* nephrotoxicity develops only with the comparatively sequestered and reactive ones, which acylate these carriers and cause irreversible injury to substrate uptake. We tested this hypothesis by measuring respiration with succinate and the uptake of succinate in mitochondria exposed in situ to cephaloridine [11], cephaloglycin [12], or imipenem [13], all of which are nephrotoxic.

The antibiotics were injected intravenously into rabbits, in doses of 300 mg/kg BW, 1 or 2 hours before sacrifice. All three toxic beta-lactams reduced respiration significantly, although cephaloglycin was the most toxic per mg dosage. All three nephrotoxins also decreased mitochondrial succinate uptake, again most severely in the case of cephaloglycin. This fits with the approximately 1.5-fold greater toxicity of cephaloglycin in producing tubular necrosis than the other two beta-lactams (Table 1). Succinate efflux was unaffected by any of the three antibiotics, indicating that reduced net uptake was the result of decreased substrate entry (Figure 3).

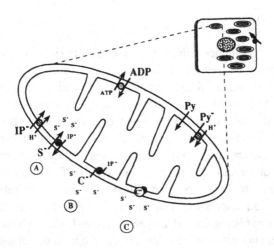

Figure 3. Proposed effects of nephrotoxic beta-lactam antibiotics on renal tubular mitochondrial function. (A) Normally, inorganic phosphate (IP$^-$) is symported into the inner mitochondrial matrix with a hydrogen ion (H$^+$) and then antiported in exchange for a metabolic sustrate such as succinate (S$^-$). (B) The nephrotoxic beta-lactams (shown here as C$^-$ for cephalosporin) fit the anionic substrate carrier, inhibiting its transport. (C) They then acylate and thereby inactivate the transporter, resulting in irreversible injury to substrate uptake and thus to mitochondrial respiration. The uptakes of phosphate, ADP and pyruvate (Py$^-$), which enter the mitochondrion by separate mechanisms, are unaffected.

Further studies tested this hypothesis by examining the specificity of the association of reduced substrate transport and reduced respiration [16]. Using succinate as the most affected substrate, we examined, first, transport and respiration after other insults to the mitochondrion; next, the organ specificity of injury in studies of liver as well as kidney mitochondria; and, finally, molecular target specificity by evaluating the effects of beta-lactam intoxication on other mitochondrial functions.

Compared to cephaloridine, cephaloglycin, and imipenem, the other potential or real mitochondrial insults studied produced different patterns of damage. Cephalexin had no inhibitory effect on uptake or respiration; respiratory chain poisons reduced respiration but did not reduce succinate uptake; although ischemia reduced both uptake and respiration, unlike the nephrotoxic beta-lactams, it also caused a large increase of succinate efflux. Measurements of mitochondrial function in another organ, the liver, showed no effect of cephaloridine or cephaloglycin on either function. Finally, studies of the effects of cephaloridine and cephaloglycin intoxication on other mitochondrial targets showed normalcy of three important functions (Figure 3). Respiration with pyruvate, which enters the mitochondrion by simple diffusion or by a proton-pyruvate symporter, was not reduced, and the uptake and efflux of phosphate and ADP, which are carried into the mitochondrion by their own transporters, were also unaffected.

Therapeutic considerations

Probably as a result of their widely varying tubular cell uptake and acylating potentials, the beta-lactams have a wide spectrum of nephrotoxic potential. With most of the commercially available beta-lactams, several of which are potentially nephrotoxic, clinical toxicity is likely to occur only under conditions of risk. As a result, the magnitude of the problem can be underestimated. These factors might explain why the nephrotoxicity of the beta-lactams has not received the attention given to that of the aminoglycosides. However, the trend toward displacement of the aminoglycosides by the newer broad-spectrum beta-lactams, and the continuing occurrence of nephrotoxicity in some of the newly released cephalosporins and the penems or thienamycins, calls for increased attention to this issue.

As a minimum, therefore, one should not assume that beta-lactam antibiotics can be used without regard to nephrotoxic potential. The clinician will want to focus upon three areas of potential prevention: (1) proper selection and administration of the antibiotics (although selection is not easy because the results of pre-release toxicologic screening are often not published); (2) recognition of documented potentiating factors (older age, decreased cardiac and/or renal function, combined use with aminoglycosides, obstructive uropathy, renal ischemia, and endotoxemia); and (3) dose adjustment where the clinical situation warrants (for example, where renal function is compromised). Transport inhibitors may be protective.

However, they should probably be avoided, because they may raise blood levels and increase toxicity if discontinued too soon.

The pharmaceutical industry can minimize the risk of nephrotoxicity by developing new beta-lactams either with limited secretory uptake by the tubular cell or with antibacterial potency derived from factors other than high reactivity. As an alternative, when a valuable antibiotic like imipenem is developed, having both rapid tubular secretion and a high acylating potential, it can be combined with an inhibitor of toxicity. Imipenem is marketed in a fixed combination with cilastatin, which blocks both its enzymatic breakdown by the kidney and its nephrotoxicity [5]. Cilastatin also appears to reduce the secretory transport of imipenem, which could explain its protective effect [5]. However, we have recently found *in vitro* protection of the mitochondrion by cilastatin (unpublished data), which suggests that it is preventing toxicity at the molecular level. This inhibitor may therefore provide the model for development of direct antagonists of beta-lactam-induced nephrotoxicity.

Acknowledgements

This work was supported by research grants from the National Institutes of Health (DK 33814) and the American Heart Association (890665), with funds contributed by the Northern California Heart Association.

References

1. Atkinson RM, Currie JP, Davis B, Pratt, DAH, Sharpe HM, Tomich EG, 1966: Acute toxicity of cephaloridine, an antibiotic derived from cephalosporin C. Toxicol Appl Pharmacol 8: 398–406.
2. Foord RD, 1975: Cephaloridine, cephalothin and the kidney. J Antimicrob Chemother 1(Suppl): 119–33.
3. Wells JS, 1972: Pharmacology and toxicology of cephalosporins, in Cephalosporins and penicillins, EH Flynn (ed). Academic Press, New York, pp. 584–608.
4. Bendirdjian J-P, Prime DJ, Browning MC, Hsu C-Y, Tune BM, 1981: Additive nephrotoxicity of cephalosporins and aminoglycosides in the rabbit. J Pharmacol Exper Therap 218: 681–5.
5. Birnbaum J, Kahan FM, Kropp H, MacDonald JS, 1985: Carbapenems. A new class of beta-lactam antibiotics. Discovery and improvement of imipenem/cilastatin. Amer J Med 78(suppl 6A): 3–21.
6. Tune BM, 1986: The nephrotoxicity of cephalosporin antibiotics – Structure-activity relationships. Comments Toxicol 1: 145–70.

7. Klastersky J, Hensgens C, Debusscher L, 1975: Empiric therapy for cancer patients: Comparative study of ticarcillin-tobramycin, ticarcillin-cephalothin, and cephalothin-tobramycin. Antimicrob Ag Chemother 7: 640–5.

8. Wade JD, Petty BG, Conrad G, Smith CR, Lipsky JJ, Ellner J, Lietman PS, 1978: Cephalothin plus an aminoglycoside is more nephrotoxic than methicillin plus an aminoglycoside. Lancet 2: 604–6.

9. The EORTC International Antimicrobial Therapy Project Group, 1978: Three antibiotic regimens in the treatment of infection in febrile granulocytopenic patients with cancer. J Infect Dis 137: 14–29.

10. Tune BM, Hsu C-Y, 1986: Augmentation of antibiotic nephrotoxicity by endotoxemia in the rabbit. J Pharmacol Exper Therap 234: 425–30.

11. Tune BM, Fravert D, Hsu C-Y, 1989: The oxidative and mitochondrial toxic effects of cephalosporin antibiotics in the kidney. A comparative study of cephaloridine and cephaloglycin. Biochem Pharmacol 38: 795–802.

12. Tune BM, Sibley RK, Hsu C-Y, 1988: The mitochondrial respiratory toxicity of cephalosporin antibiotics. An inhibitory effect on substrate uptake. J Pharmacol Exper Therap 245: 1054–9.

13. Tune BM, Fravert D, Hsu C-Y, 1989: Thienamycin nephrotoxicity: Mitochondrial injury and oxidative effects of imipenem in the rabbit kidney. Biochem Pharmacol, 38: 3779–3783.

14. Indelicato JM, Dinner A, Peters LR, Wilham WL, 1977: Hydrolysis of 3-chloro-3-cephems. Intramolecular nucleophilic attack in cefaclor. J Med Chem 20: 961–3.

15. Bendirdjian J-P, Prime DJ, Browning MC, Tune BM, 1982: The mitochondrial respiratory toxicity of cephalosporins. Molecular properties and pathogenic significance, in Nephrotoxicity, Ototoxicity of Drugs. J-P Fillastre (ed). Editions IN-SERM, Rouen, pp. 303–19.

16. Tune BM, Hsu C-Y, 1990: The renal mitochondrial toxicity of cephalosporins: Specificity of the effect on anionic substrate uptake. J Pharmacol Exper Therap, 252: 65–69.

Prevention of analgesic nephropathy

ULRICH C. DUBACH

Clinical evidence that analgesic use or abuse causes analgesic nephropathy relies on the association from retrospective clinical or autopsy surveys and on prospective case control studies. The incidence of analgesic nephropathy shows geographical differences. The nephrotoxicity of analgesics may also be influenced by local factors such as fluid intake, consumption of other drugs, environmental conditions, and genetic factors. The principal risk appears to be the level of analgesic use and specific abuse. Abuse of analgesics, nearly always in combination products, is related to their use to reduce strain and increase productivity in a working environment. It is predominantly women in their thirties and forties with disturbed backgrounds and who show signs of personality or psychiatric disorders, who abuse analgesics. In most cases, the analgesics are taken for rather ill-defined tension headaches and migraine, insomnia, depression, and agitation rather than for more defined painful conditions. The incorporation in analgesic combinations of drugs with mood altering and/or analgesic effects, such as shown with phenacetin, codeine, and caffeine, leads to habituation and, therefore, to excessive use and abuse.

It must be remembered that the spotlight has always been on phenacetin since it was first described in 1953 in Switzerland. It has, however, always been taken in combination with other analgesics. It was phenacetin that was subsequently restricted in availability or banned in a number of countries, although its withdrawal has not been followed in some countries by the expected reduction in the incidence of analgesic-associated nephropathy. Today, the abuse of analgesics and the development of the nephropathy is overwhelmingly linked to the ingestion of combination products. Abusers only rarely take single drug products, and epidemiological studies have shown that analgesic nephropathy associated with one single drug is very rare. It is not surprising that tighter regulations for phenacetin or its removal

M. E. De Broe and G. A. Verpooten (eds.): Prevention in Nephrology, 51–53.
© 1991 Kluwer Academic Publishers. Printed in the Netherlands.

from the market by health authorities has not influenced the incidence of analgesic nephropathy in various countries. A combination product which is left on the market where phenacetin is replaced by paracetamol, still appears to represent a risk for the development of analgesic nephropathy in those who abuse analgesics. Therefore, calls and recommendations for tighter control of their availability in those countries which still represent a significant problem, have been heard. The countries especially involved are Switzerland, Belgium, Denmark, West Germany, The Netherlands, and some regions in the USA. Strict regulations against combination analgesics are already enforced in Australia but, again, these do not, as yet, seem to have reduced the rate of analgesic nephropathy up to 1985. A certain fall in the incidence of renal disease in some countries may not, therefore, be attributed alone to the removal of phenacetin: analgesic nephropathy continues to be a problem, even where phenacetin has been removed from OTC sales!

Effect of restriction on analgesic use

In 1961 in Sweden and Denmark and in 1965 in Finland, phenacetin was restricted to prescription only. In Sweden, the consumption of phenacetin containing tablets fell from 31.4 million in 1959 to 1.8 million in 1962. Deaths from uremia in analgesic abusers showed no fall over the following five years, but the incidence of analgesic nephropathy has fallen since then to a point where it is now rarely seen in these countries. Phenacetin was removed from many of the OTC mixtures and compounds in 1962 in Australia, although the two most popular brands retained it as part of their formula until 1967 in one case and 1975 in the other. In 1977, the "Mixed Analgesic Legislation" was introduced which restricted OTC analgesics to one single substance and combined analgesics were only available thereafter on prescription. Despite these measures, there has been little fall-off in renal failure attributed to analgesic nephropathy. In Canada, restrictions were placed on phenacetin in 1972 and it was removed from the market entirely in 1975, but by 1978, the incidence of renal disease had not declined, although later estimates in 1982 indicated a 50% reduction.

Both the Swedish and Canadian experiences suggest a considerable lag period before restrictions in availability are reflected in reductions in incidence, even if the two are related. There have been major improvements in the treatment of renal disease and the complications over the last 20 years and, furthermore, the heightened public awareness campaigns in some countries may have helped to reduce analgesic abuse over the same period.

Recommendations

The 1984 report of the "Antwerp Nephropathy Project" presented very valuable suggestions from many experts in the field on preventive methods which could be undertaken to reduce the abuse of OTC analgesics. Similarly, in 1984, the US National Institute of Health convinced a consensus development conference on analgesic-associated kidney diseases to consider the problem. The most important conclusions were: the introduction of educational programs, the restriction of OTC sale to single analgesics only, prescription for combination analgesics, the restriction of pack sizes, the removal of compounds with mood-altering effects (codeine, caffeine, barbiturates), restrictive advertising to pain relieving properties only, and continued research on analgesic abuse.

Efficacy and nephrotoxicity of aminoglycosides

H. MATTIE

Because of their nephrotoxicity, aminoglycosides have been the subject of intensive study for many years. They are indeed an important cause of acute impairment of renal function which is why they have received so much attention from nephrologists. However, before discussing measures that may help to diminish the impact of aminoglycoside nephrotoxicity, this phenomenon should be seen in the proper perspective. The renal toxicity induced by the administration of aminoglycosides is a minor problem: the incidence is low and the condition is practically always reversible. The destruction of the hair cells of cochlea and vestibulum has led to much more human suffering, especially because this effect is often irreversible; several patients have become completely deaf after aminoglycoside therapy. Ototoxicity is therefore the main reason why plasma concentrations of aminoglycosides must remain as low as possible: in fact the usefulness of aminoglycosides as life-saving antibiotics is severely limited because of this aspect [1]. In this respect, impaired renal function is also an important risk factor for ototoxicity. Since aminoglycoside nephrotoxicity is probably also concentration-dependent, control of plasma concentrations should not only help to protect the kidneys but also the inner ear.

In this short review, the mechanisms of the renal toxicity of amino-glycosides, together with the possibility of counteracting this effect, will be discussed. In addition, the relation between antibiotic efficacy and nephrotoxicity, i.e. the therapeutic window of the aminoglycosides, will also be considered.

The main site of the aminoglycoside nephrotoxic effect is the proximal tubular cell [2]. The concentration to which these cells are exposed from the luminal side is approximately equal to the plasma concentration. Since toxicity is usually concentration-dependent, monitoring of plasma concentrations is essential for a study of aminoglycoside toxicity. Although amino-

M. E. De Broe and G. A. Verpooten (eds.): Prevention in Nephrology, 55–63.

glycosides are highly polar drugs – and therefore do not pass easily through cellular membranes – it has been shown that they can enter the tubular cell by a process which involves binding to negative charges on the brush border and pinocytosis [3]. Once inside the cell, the aminoglycosides exert their toxic effect which, in the end, leads to cell destruction.

The relative importance of various toxic effects, such as enzyme inhibition, is as yet unknown. The most conspicuous histological feature, however, is the uptake of aminoglycosides in lysosomes [4], leading to the development of so-called myeloid bodies. These changes occur early, before the impairment of renal function [4, 5], and will lead to cell death, even after administration of the drug has ceased.

During treatment, however, regeneration already occurs [6] and the newly formed tubular cells seem to exhibit greater resistance to the aminoglycosides. This may be one of the reasons why clinically important impairment of renal function is a relatively rare event. For the same reason, the incidence of nephrotoxicity found in various clinical studies is probably a gross underestimate of tubular damage, since it only represents the net result of cell necrosis and regeneration.

Moreover, the criteria used to define renal impairment in most clinical trials are often relatively insensitive. This is illustrated by Figure 1, which shows the parameters of renal function used in a comparative trial of tobramycin and netilmicin [7]. According to commonly used criteria, none of the patients suffered renal impairment. (Note that comparison of the absolute changes in serum creatinine in the two groups of patients demonstrates with much more statistical sensitivity that there was indeed no difference between the two aminoglycosides in their effect on creatinine clearance during the acute phase and in the long run.)

In experimental animals, regeneration of tubular cells is clearly age-dependent [8], which may explain why age has turned out to be a risk factor for renal toxicity in man. This may not be the whole truth, however, since in that situation many factors that might influence aminoglycoside nephrotoxicity are closely correlated. For instance, the correlation between age and renal function makes it difficult to distinguish between the two in severely ill patients, and if creatinine is used as a parameter of renal function, it is self-evident that at a given serum creatinine level, renal function will be less in an elderly patient than in a young patient [8]. In this respect, the analysis by Moore et al. [9] is still outstanding, since these authors applied stepwise discriminant analysis to their data. Their results indicate that high aminoglycoside concentrations in plasma, in particular

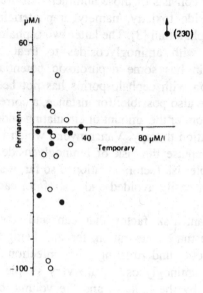

Figure 1. Change in serum creatinine under treatment with tobramycin (o) or netilmicin (•). The temporary change is expressed as the difference between the maximum concentration during treatment and the minimum initial value. The permanent change is the difference between the ultimate concentration and the concentration before treatment.

maximum concentrations, are an important risk factor. Less easy to explain is why they also found hepatic disorder and female sex as risk factors. As a matter of fact, in animal experiments, the latter findings could not be confirmed [10, 11].

Another possible risk factor is the simultaneous administration of other nephrotoxic drugs. For this reason, it is recommended that patients should not receive aminoglycosides for an infection if they have been treated, are being treated, or will be treated for cancer with *cis*-platinum [8]. Of course, it is just as rational to discourage the use of *cis*-platinum in patients who have recently undergone aminoglycoside therapy, but for obvious reasons, this advice is seldom heard.

Methoxyflurane and furosemide are also supposed to enhance amino-glycoside nephrotoxicity [8]. Cyclosporin A, a recently introduced im-munosuppressive drug, can be nephrotoxic. However, since the site of its toxic action is clearly different from that of the aminoglycosides [12], it is not really certain that the two types of drug are incompatible.

A special category consists of those antimicrobial drugs that are said to enhance aminoglycoside toxicity, namely amphotericin B, clindamycin, cephaloridine, and cephalothin [8]. The latter two cephalosporins have often been used together with aminoglycosides to treat serious infections; moreover, cephalothin has some nephrotoxic potential on its own. In animals an interaction with cephalosporins has not been confirmed, and other explanations are also possible: for instance, a correlation between the severity of the infection, or the amount of circulating endotoxin, and the use of antibiotic combination therapy. Vancomycin, which is also nephrotoxic, does not seem to increase the risk of aminoglycoside toxicity [13, 14]. Looking at the possible risk factors mentioned so far, it should be clear that most of them are not easily avoided and, therefore, cannot play a role in preventive measures.

The most important risk factor that can and, therefore, should be monitored, is the plasma concentration, the aim being to avoid excessive concentrations without undertreating the infection [15]. The pharmacokinetics of the aminoglycosides are very simple, since the drug is excreted exclusively by the kidneys and the volume of distribution corresponds to that of extracellular water. For practical reasons, most nomograms or computer programs lead to the calculation of a reliable initial dosage schedule, based on body weight and creatinine clearance, whether measured or predicted [16]. Nevertheless, it is generally agreed that actual concentrations have to be measured as a check on the calculations and that renal function should be assessed frequently. It is more difficult to agree on the plasma concentrations required for patients with impaired renal function.

Most programs aim at the maximum tolerated peak concentrations as well as the maximum tolerated trough levels. This will often lead to an increase in mean plasma concentrations in patients with impaired renal function and, thereby, probably to increased toxicity. One solution would be to further decrease the dose, but it is difficult to assess how that would affect efficacy. As a result, this approach is seldom applied.

The next question is whether specific measures can be used to counteract the nephrotoxicity of aminoglycosides. Although considerable experimental work has been devoted to this question, most of the results of these investigations are not easily applicable in clinical practice. Since entry of aminoglycosides into the tubular cell depends on the polarity of the drug, the effect of several anions and cations has been investigated. Bicarbonates, and acetazolamide seem to offer some protection in animal experiments

[17]. This is at least a feasible approach for patients, but, as yet, its possible usefulness has not been evaluated. It should be noted in this respect that the antibacterial efficacy of aminoglycosides is also dependent on pH and ionic strength. Therefore, the measures that might diminish toxicity could also be detrimental to efficacy, especially in urinary tract infections. Free radicals have been suggested as a factor responsible for the toxic effects of aminoglycosides; in fact scavengers such as dimethyl thiourea, dimethylsulfoxide, and deferoxamine had a protective effect in rats [18], whereas tocopherol did not [19]. Angiotensin-converting enzyme inhibitors may protect against renal vasoconstriction induced by gentamicin [20], although this finding could not be confirmed by others [21]. Anyhow, the possible consequences of this finding for the prevention of clinical nephrotoxicity have not been investigated.

It would appear that the best way to prevent aminoglycoside toxicity is to avoid using aminoglycosides. Currently, the pharmaceutical industry seems to be working towards the goal of making aminoglycosides superfluous; clinical trials have been performed to prove that serious infections can be treated without aminoglycosides [22]. At present, the antibacterial spectra of third-generation cephalosporins, as well as the fluoroquinolones, are such that aminoglycosides are no longer needed for many infections. Nevertheless, aminoglycosides are still widely used for initial empirical therapy in combination with beta-lactam antibiotics. If the patient improves on this combination, aminoglycoside therapy is often continued, even after the causative micro-organism has been shown to be sensitive to the other antibiotic, thus disregarding the evidence that monotherapy with, for instance, a third generation cephalosporin is not inferior to that with the combination. Moreover, it is often not realized that the maximum tolerated dose is not required in all instances; for example, in the case of very sensitive organisms or a synergistic combination with penicillin for treatment of an enterococcal infection, a dose much lower than the conventional one would do as well.

If, however, it is necessary to administer aminoglycosides in their maximum effective dosages, then the questions are what is the least toxic aminoglycoside and what is the least toxic dosage schedule? Obviously, these questions are directly related to two other questions: what is the most potent aminoglycoside and what is the most effective dosage schedule. So far, an unequivocal answer has not been found.

There is considerable direct and indirect data on the comparative nephrotoxicities of the various aminoglycoside antibiotics. With respect to cortical uptake and tubular cell damage, gentamicin is probably the most nephrotoxic of the aminoglycosides in use today; tobramycin and netilmicin are less nephrotoxic and amikacin even less toxic [23, 24].

It is not at all clear that this also holds for ototoxicity, which should remain the overriding concern in terms of danger for the patient. Unfortunately, comparison of the aminoglycosides – especially in clinical trials – has most often been carried out at fixed dosage levels, so that it is impossible to quantitate the relative toxicities. In other words, if netilmicin is less nephrotoxic than gentamicin, how much less toxic is it? For this reason, it is still difficult to compare relative toxicity with relative efficacy. Animal experiments indicate that the relative efficacy of aminoglycosides in vivo is reflected fairly accurately by the relative efficacy in vitro, but the existing differences in efficacy between aminoglycosides are not apparent in the recommended dosage schedules. In the case, for instance, of an infection with Pseudomonas aeruginosa, the efficacy of tobramycin against this particular micro-organism is twice that of gentamicin or netilmicin. Since the recommended doses of tobramycin and gentamicin are similar, tobramycin should offer the most favourable therapeutic index of the two for this kind of infection. Comparison of tobramycin and netilmicin is actually more complex, since the recommended dose of netilmicin is 50% higher than that of tobramycin, while its anti-Pseudomonas activity is only half that of tobramycin.

In other words, the two antibiotics have never been compared clinically in equi-effective dosages [25]. Once a particular aminoglycoside has been chosen on the basis of its therapeutic index, its optimal dosage schedule should be established. In this respect, toxicological arguments are more compelling than those on efficacy: in general, it is agreed that many divided doses are more toxic than larger doses administered at longer intervals [26, 27]. Like the comparison of different aminoglycosides, a comparison of different dosage schedules for a particular total daily dose has not been performed; therefore it has only been shown that a certain daily dose is less toxic when given as a single dose than when given in divided dosages, but not how much less toxic. The probable explanation for the greater toxicity of a divided dose is that in the range of therapeutic concentrations, the uptake of aminoglycosides in tubular cells is a saturable process [28]. Therefore, the total daily tubular uptake would be less if the daily dose is given as a single dose than when given as divided dosages.

Unfortunately, most physicians feel uneasy about treating infectious diseases with large doses of antibiotics given at long intervals, notwithstanding accumulating evidence that, as far as aminoglycosides are concerned, this would not be detrimental to the patient. At least single large doses may be no less effective than many divided doses. The reasons for this are several. Aminoglycosides have in vitro a rapidly killing effect; this effect is not only dose dependent but even at relatively high concentrations the maximum killing rate of aminoglycosides is not yet observed. This killing rate in vitro is proportional to the logarithm of the concentration [29]. In vivo, the concentration declines exponentially; combining these two conditions mathematically it could be predicted that the efficacy of amino-glycosides in vivo will be proportional to the area under the logarithm of the concentration curve (Mattie *et al.*, to be published), as was confirmed by the results of experimental infections [30].

Although these results are not identical with the hypothesis that the same daily dose has the same effect, irrespective of the dosage schedule, quantitatively they are not much different. Therefore, clinical studies aimed at solving this issue are justified. One problem in planning such clinical trials is that, for practical reasons, the administration of only one daily dosage is aimed at, and it is difficult to extrapolate from the animal experiments whether in man a 24-hour interval would not be too long. The results of at least one recent clinical trial suggest that a 24-hour interval is, indeed, too long [31]: in a subgroup of patients with urinary tract infections, the success rate in patients receiving one daily dose was only 58%, while in patients receiving divided dosages, it was 81%. Although this difference did not reach the level of significance, it was still large enough to be a source of concern. After all, the burden of proof is still on those advocating one daily dosage and not on those who, from the point of view of efficacy, want to stay with two or three daily dosages.

To summarize, the following conclusions can be drawn, all of which should be considered with caution:

- toxicity is the most important drawback in the use of aminoglycosides;
- ototoxicity is more serious than nephrotoxicity;
- practically speaking, there are no nontoxic dosage levels [32];
- toxicity can be minimized by giving the lowest possible dose for the shortest possible time;
- the total daily dose should not be divided too often;
- the aminoglycoside with the highest therapeutic index is the drug-of-choice.

62

And, finally:

– the only way to avoid aminoglycoside toxicity entirely is not to administer aminoglycosides.

References

1. Lerner SA, Matz GJ, Hawkins JE Jr. (eds), 1984: Aminoglycoside ototoxicity. Little, Brown, Boston.
2. Kaloyanidis GJ, 1984: Renal pharmacology of aminoglycoside antibiotics, in Kidney, small proteins and drugs. Bianchi C, Bertelli A, Duarte CG (eds). Karger, Basel, pp. 148–67.
3. Collier VU, Lietman PS, Mitch WE, 1979: Evidence for luminal uptake of gentamicin in the perfused rat kidney. J Pharmacol Exp Ther 210: 247–51.
4. De Broe ME, Paulus GJ, Verpooten GA et al., 1984: Early effects of gentamicin, tobramycin, and amikacin on the human kidney. Kidney Int 25: 643–52.
5. Tulkens PM, 1984: Aminoglycoside nephrotoxicity: recent insights and perspectives, in Kidney, small proteins and drugs. Bianchi C, Bertelli A, Duarte CG (eds). Karger, Basel, pp. 168–81.
6. Giuliano RA, Paulus GJ, Verpooten GA et al., 1984: Recovery of cortical phospholipidosis and necrosis after acute gentamicin loading in rats. Kidney Int 26: 838–47.
7. Mattie H, 1981: in Current concepts in aminoglycoside therapy. Michel MF (ed). Excerpta Medica, Amsterdam, Oxford, Princeton, pp. 37–40.
8. Humes HD, O'Connor RP, 1988: Aminoglycoside nephrotoxicity, in Diseases of the kidney. Schrier RW, Gottschalk CW (eds). Little, Brown, Boston, Toronto, pp. 1229–73.
9. Moore RD, Smith CR, Lipsky TJ, Mellits ED, Lietman PS, 1984: Risk factors for nephrotoxicity in patients treated with aminoglycosides. Ann Int Med 100: 352–7.
10. Camps J, Sola X, Rimola A et al., 1988: Comparative study of aminoglycoside nephrotoxicity in normal rats and rats with experimental cirrhosis. Hepatology 8: 837–44.
11. Bayliss C, 1989: Gentamicin-induced glomerulotoxicity in the pregnant rat. Am J Kidney Disease 13: 108–13.
12. Bennett WM, 1986: Comparison of cyclosporine nephrotoxicity with aminoglycoside nephrotoxicity. Clinical Nephrology 25 Suppl 1, S126–9.
13. Kacew S, Hewitt WR, Hook JB, 1989: Gentamicin-induced renal metabolic alterations in newborn rat kidney: lack of potentiation by vancomycin. Toxicol App Pharmacol 99: 61–71.
14. Cimino MA, Rotstein C, Slaughter RL, Emrich LJ, 1987: Relationship of serum antibiotic concentrations to nephrotoxicity in cancer patients receiving concurrent aminoglycoside and vancomycin therapy. Am J Med 83: 1091–7.
15. Mattie H, Craig WA, Pechère JC, 1989: Determinants of efficacy and toxicity of aminoglycosides. J Antimicrob Chemother 24: 281–95.

16. Hallynck T, Soep HH, Thomis J, Boelaert J, Daneels R, Fillastre JP, De Rosa F, Rubinstein E, Hatala M, Spousta J, Dettli L, 1981: Prediction of creatinine clearance from serum creatinine concentration based on lean body mass. Clin Pharmacol Ther 30: 414–21.

17. Aynedjian HS, Nguyen D, Lee HY, Sablay LB, Bank N, 1988: Effects of dietary electrolyte supplementation on gentamicin nephrotoxicity. Am J Med Sci 295: 442–52.

18. Walker PD, Shah SV, 1988: Evidence suggesting a role for hydroxyl radical in gentamicin-induced acute renal failure in rats. J Clin Invest 81: 334–41.

19. Ramsammy LS, Josepovitz C, Ling KY, Lane BD, Kaloyanides GJ, 1987: Failure of inhibition of lipid peroxidation by vitamin E to protect against gentamicin nephrotoxicity in the rat. Biochem Pharmacol 36: 2125–32.

20. Schor N, Ichikawa I, Rennke HG, Troy JL, Brenner BM, 1981: Pathophysiology of altered glomerular function in aminoglycoside-treated rats. Kidney Int 19: 288–96.

21. Luft FC, Aronoff GR, Evan AP, Connors BA, Weinberger MH, Kleit SA, 1982: The renin-angiotensin system in aminoglycoside-induced acute renal failure. J Pharmacol Exp Ther 220: 433–9.

22. Lagast H, Klastersky J, Kains JP, Van der Auwera P, Meunier F, Woussen F, Thijs JP, 1986: Empiric therapy with aztreonam or ceftazidime in gram-negative septicemia. Am J Med 80 Suppl 5C: 79–84.

23. Soberon L, Bowman RL, Pastoriza-Munoz E, Kaloyanides GJ, 1979: Comparative nephrotoxicities of gentamicin, netilmicin and tobramycin in the rat. J Pharmacol Exp Ther 210: 334–43.

24. Fillastre JP, Hemet J, Tulkens P et al., 1983: Comparative nephrotoxicity of four amino-glycosides: biochemical and ultrastructural modifications of lysosomes. Adv Nephrol 12: 253–75.

25. Lerner AM, Reyes MP, Cone LA et al., 1983: Randomised, controlled trial of the comparative efficacy, auditory toxicity, and nephrotoxicity of tobramycin and netilmicin. Lancet ii: 1123–7.

26. Giuliano RA, Verpooten GA, De Broe ME, 1986: The effect of dosing strategy on kidney cortical accumulation of aminoglycosides in rats. Am J Kidney Diseases 8: 297–303.

27. Verpooten GA, Giuliano RA, Verbist L, Eestermans G, De Broe ME, 1989: Once-daily dosing decreases renal accumulation of gentamicin and netilmicin. Clin Pharmacol Ther 45: 22–7.

28. Giuliano RA, Verpooten GA, Verbist L, Wedeen RP, De Broe ME, 1986: In vivo uptake kinetics of aminoglycosides in the kidney cortex of rats. J Pharmacol Exp Ther 236: 470–5.

29. Hoogeterp JJ, Mattie H, Terporten P, 1988: The relative efficacies of tobramycin and ciprofloxacin against Pseudomonas aeruginosa in vitro and in normal and granulocytopenic mice. Infection 16: 58–62.

30. Vogelman B, Gudmundsson S, Leggett J, Turnidge J, Ebert S, Craig WA, 1988: Correlation of antimicrobial pharmacokinetic parameters with therapeutic efficacy in an animal model. J Inf Dis 158: 831–47.

31. Sturm AW, 1989: Netilmicin in the treatment of gram-negative bacteremia: single daily versus multiple daily dosage. J Inf Dis 159: 931–7.

32. MacDougall ML, 1988: Aminoglycosides antibiotics: unsafe at any dose? J Lab Clin Med 112: 669–70.

Prevention of cadmium and lead nephropathy

RICHARD P. WEDEEN

Lead and cadmium nephropathy are rarely identified outside of the occupational setting, but the frequency of diagnosis may not reflect the prevalence of disease. Standardized diagnostic criteria for these renal diseases are not available and end-stage renal disease registries make no provision for their identification. Determining the etiology of chronic renal disease is difficult when causation is multifactorial and the attack rate is low. Moreover, the diagnostic effort may seem unjustified when the pathologic process is irreversible. It has long been suspected that environmental toxins produce renal damage but since long-term, low-level exposure leaves neither specific physical findings nor historical clues, physicians are usually unable to determine etiology in individual patients. Yet etiologic diagnosis is essential if prevention is to be achieved.

Clinicians must use epidemiologic tools if they wish to control the exorbitant costs of therapeutic "half-way technologies"; dialysis and transplantation. They must look beyond the simple causal concepts of the germ theory if prevention is to play a role in Nephrology. Prevention may have to be undertaken despite multifactorial etiology and consequent uncertainty concerning causality. Failure to do so errs on the side of disease promotion.

Occupational kidney disease provides a model for identifying environmental kidney disease [1]. Lead and cadmium have been implicated in the production of slowly progressive, chronic interstitial nephritis in humans (Table 1; [2–4]). These environmental nephrotoxins are unique because they are stored in the body for decades; lead in the skeleton, cadmium in liver and kidney. Tissue storage reflects a sumation of net past absorption and therefore is more useful than urine or blood for estimating cumulative exposure. High levels of lead exposure have been associated with the interstitial nephritis of gout sometimes referred to as gouty nephropathy

M. E. De Broe and G. A. Verpooten (eds.): Prevention in Nephrology. 65–72.
© 1991 Kluwer Academic Publishers. Printed in the Netherlands.

Table 1. Pb v Cd nephropathy – similarities

	Pb	Cd
Renal	TIN, PT, nuclear	TIN, PT, lysosome
	Acute Fanconi	Chronic Fanconi
Latency	3–30 yrs	3–30 yrs
Storage	90% skeletal	60% liver + kid
	@ 10 yrs	@ 10 yrs
Diagnosis	in vivo XRF	in vivo XRF, NAA
Reproduction/growth	dysfunction	dysfunction

TIN = tubulointerstitial nephritis; PT = proximal tubule; XRF = X-ray fluorescence.

Table 2. Pb v Cd nephropathy – differences

	Pb	Cd
Hypertension	+	?
Gout	+	-
Neurobehavioral	+	-
Kidney stones	-	+
Osteomalacia	-	+
LMW proteinuria	-	+
Critical organ	?vascular, CNS	PT

LMW = low molecular weight; CNS = cental nervous system.

(Table 2; [3–5]). Low-level lead absorption is associated with hypertension in adults and neurobehavioral deficits in children.

Osteomalacia and nephrolithiasis, due to renal calcium wasting, produce the clinical symptoms of cadmium nephrotoxicity due to renal calcium wasting [2, 6, 7]). A high incidence of calcium stones has been found in men occupationally exposed to cadmium in Britain, Sweden and the United States. In Japan, devasting bone demineralization occurred particularly in multiparous, nutritionally deficient women environmentally exposed to cadmium from contaminated rice. The severe bone pain caused by the osteomalacia earned the name "itai-itai" or "ouch-ouch" disease.

Cadmium nephropathy is characterized by low molecular-weight proteinuria (beta-2-microglobulin, retinol binding protein, etc.) due to diminished proximal tubule uptake and metabolism of these filtered proteins. There is increasing evidence that this proximal tubular injury predicts development of renal failure in cadmium nephropathy. The mean serum creatinine concentration in 21 Japanese subjects with itai-

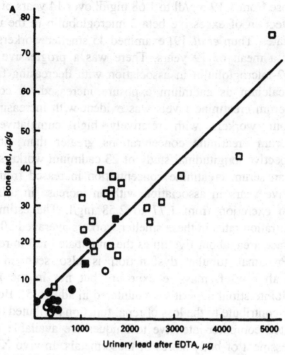

Figure 1. Correlation between chelatable lead and iliac crest bone lead concentration. (From Van de Vyver *et al.* [19] with permission.)

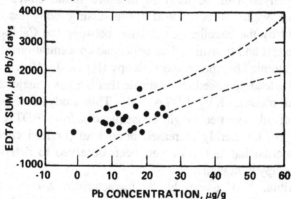

Figure 2. Relationship between tibial lead concentration (determined by in-vivo XRF) and chelatable lead. Broken lines represent 95% confidence limits of transiliac bone leads and EDTA tests in Figure 1 (above). Transiliac leads were multiplied by 1.75 to adjust for higher bone lead concentrations in tibia [11]. (From Wedeen *et al.* [16] with permission.)

itai disease rose from 1.19 mg/dl to 1.68 mg/dl over 14 years of observation following detection of excessive beta-2-microglobulin in the urine [8]. In the United States, Thun *et al.* [9] examined 45 smelter workers exposed to cadmium for a mean of 19 years. There was a progressive increase in urinary beta-2-microglobulin in association with decreasing tubular reabsorption of calcium as cadmium exposure increased. A corresponding increase in serum creatinine levels was evident with increasing cadmium exposure; four workers with relatively high cumulative exposures developed serum creatinine concentrations greater than 1.6 mg/dl. In another prospective longitudinal study of 23 cadmium workers in Belgium [10], the mean serum creatinine concentration increased from 1.2 to 1.5 mg/dl over five years in association with an increase in urinary beta-2-microglobulin excretion from 1.77 to 2.58 mg/l. The estimated fall in glomerular filtration rates in these smelter workers averaged 30 ml/min/1.73 m^2 body surface area, about five times the anticipated fall in renal function with age. Proximal tubular dysfunction is also seen in acute lead nephropathy after brief, massive exposure but not in the lead-induced chronic tubulointerstitial nephritis encountered in adults [5]. Both cadmium and lead may contribute to the loss of renal function attributed to aging.

Sophisticated computer-intensive techniques are available for the non-invasive assessment of body stores of these metals. In-vivo X-ray fluorescence (XRF) can be used for both lead and cadmium and in-vivo neutron activation analysis can be used to measure tissue stores of cadmium [11–18]. The value of bone lead for assessing body lead stores was demonstrated by the excellent correlation between the CaNa$_2$EDTA lead-mobilization test and transiliac iliac bone lead concentrations determined in biopsies by atomic absorption spectroscopy (Figure 1; [19]). Recent studies in chronically lead-poisoned rats indicate that bone is a major source of the urinary lead mobilized by EDTA [20]. This study also suggested the possibility of adverse neurologic consequences from EDTA because the chelating agent transiently increased brain lead (or lead chelate) in rats. Cerebral function has not, however, been observed to deteriorate during chelation therapy in humans.

In-vivo tibial XRF using the K characteristic X-rays of lead gives virtually the same information on bone lead as that obtained by bone biopsy (Figure 2). Both measurements average the lead over the full cortical bone thickness. Ninety-five percent of the body lead burden is retained in bone with a biological half-life approximating 10 years. The biological half-life of blood lead, on the other hand, approximates two weeks. In addition, the range of blood lead concentrations in individuals without symptoms of acute lead poisoning (colic, neuropathy, encephalopathy and anemia) is too narrow to effectively distinguish between different body burdens that are readily separated by the EDTA test or in-vivo tibial XRF. Blood lead measurements are useful for assessing recent lead absorption but may be misleading for assessing cumulative past exposure. The non-invasive XRF technique for measuring tibial lead content is safe, practical and sufficiently sensitive to detect individuals with excessive body lead burdens. XRF is likely to replace both EDTA testing and blood lead measurements in the near future.

The advantages of using K X-rays over the low energy lead L X-rays were reviewed at an international meeting convened by the United States National Institute of Environmental Health Sciences, The Environmental Protection Agency and the University of Maryland in March 1989 [21]. The conferees agreed that the tibia was the site of choice for bone lead measurements but that the calcaneous could provide special insight into lead metabolism in trabecular bone. L X-rays may provide information on the metabolism of lead in the subperiosteal 0.3 mm of bone [22]. Since lead is not distributed homogeneously from bone surface to marrow cavity in adult tibias [23], surface measurements do not reflect total bone stores. Because of the extensive soft tissue absorption, L X-rays are difficult to calibrate and highly dependent on small geometric shifts in the leg relative to the detector. K X-ray measurements, on the other hand, are largely independent of overlying soft tissue and bone geometry and can be normalized by comparison to Rayleigh scattering arising from bone calcium and phosphorus. Excellent correlations have been obtained between tibial K XRF measurements and in-vitro atomic absorption spectroscopy [16].

While occupational exposures provide the clinical foundation for recognizing renal disease arising from environmental exposure, it cannot be assumed that the relationship between blood or urine concentrations and cumulative tissue levels will be the same after low-level environmental exposure as after high-level occupational exposure. The influence of low-level lead absorption on blood pressure for example, could not be discerned in bloods from lead workers because blood lead levels were routinely high in this group [24]. The effect of lead on blood pressure revealed by epidemiologic studies occurs at much lower body lead burdens than does lead-induced renal failure in hypertensives [25]. Moreover, interactions with other environmental factors including diet may modify both the sensitivity of individuals to environmental nephrotoxins and the clinical manifestations. Similarly, the concentration of cadmium in biological fluids may have a different relationship to tissues stores after environmental as opposed to occupational exposure. A wide range of urinary cadmium has been observed in individuals with cadmium nephropathy. Urinary cadmium concentrations average only 10 mcg/g creatinine in itai-itai disease [8], while in the industrial setting, urine cadmiums of 10 mcg/g creatinine or less are considered "normal" [2].

Association alone cannot prove causation, but association is essential to establish the etiologic relationship. The first step is to show that both the heavy metal and interstitial nephritis are present. For the individual patient, high tissue lead or cadmium levels suggest etiology when other causes of renal disease have been ruled out. For the population as a whole, determining the distribution of body burdens of lead and cadmium is necessary to calculate the relative risk for kidney disease from specific exposure levels. Linear regression analysis can indicate the relative contribution of different potential etiologic factors when the renal disease is multifactorial. When risk ratios are calculated from epidemiologic data, compelling arguments can be presented to control environmental pollution in order to prevent renal disease. Only then can the cost of kidney disease be weighed against the economic value of introducing these metals into the environment.

References

1. Wedeen RP, 1988: Occupational and environmental renal diseases. Curr Nephro 11: 65–106.
2. Kjellstrom T, 1986: Renal effects, in Cadmium and health: A toxicological and epidemiological appraisal. Friberg L, Elinder C-G, Kjellstrom T, Nordberg GF (eds). CRC Press, Boca Raton, Vol II, pp. 21–110.
3. Batuman V, Maesaka JK, Haddad B, Tepper E, Landy E, Wedeen RP, 1981: The role of lead in gout nephropathy. N Engl J Med 304: 520–3.
4. Ritz E, Mann J, Stoeppler M, 1988: Lead and the kidney, Adv Nephrol 17: 241–74.
5. Wedeen RP, 1984: Poison in the pot: The legacy of lead. Southern Illinois University Press, Carbondale.
6. Nicaud P, Lafitte A, Gross A, 1942: Les troubles de l'intoxication chronique par le cadmium. Arch Mal Prof Med 1: 192–202.
7. Scott R, Cunningham C, McLelland A, 1982: The importance of cadmium as a factor in calcified upper urinary tract stone disease: A prospective 7-year study. Br J Urol 54:584–9.
8. Kido T, Nogawa K, Ishizaki M, Honda R, Tsuritani I, Yamada Y, Nakagawa A, 1990: Long-term observation of serum creatinine and arterial blood pH in persons with

cadmium-induced renal dysfunction, Arch Environ Health 45: 35–41.

9. Thun MJ, Osorio AM, Schober S, Hannon WH, Halperin W, 1989: Nephropathy in cadmium workers – Assessment of risk from airborne occupational cadmium exposure. Br J Ind Med 46: 689–697.

10. Roels HA, Lauwerys RR, Buchet JP, Bernard AM, Vos A, Oversteyns M, 1989: Health significance of cadmium-induced renal dysfunction: A five-year follow-up. Brit J Indust Med 46: 755–64.

11. Ahlgren L, Mattson S, 1981: Cadmium in man measured in vivo by X-ray fluorescence analysis. Phys Med Biol 26: 19–26.

12. Chettle DR, Franklin DM, Guthrie CJG, Scott MC, Somervaille LJ, 1987: In-vivo and in-vitro measurements of lead and cadmium. Biol Trace Element Res 13: 191–208.

13. Scott MC, Chettle DR, 1986: In-vivo elemental analysis in experimental medicine, Scand J Work Environ Health 12: 81–96.

14. Roels HA, Lauwerys RR, Buchet J-P, Bernard A, Chettle DR, Harvey TC, Al-Haddad IK, 1981: In vivo measurement of liver and kidney cadmium in workers exposed to this metal: Its significance with respect to cadmium in blood and urine. Environ Res 26: 217–40.

15. Jones KW, Schlidlovksy G, Williams FH, Wedeen RP, Batuman V, 1987: In vivo determination of tibial lead by K X-ray fluorescence with a Cd-109 source, in In vivo body composition studies. Ellis KJ, Yamamura S, Morgan WD (eds). Institute of Physical Sciences in Medicine, London, pp. 363–73.

16. Wedeen RP, Batuman V, Quinless F, Williams FH Jr, Bogden J, Schlidovsky G, Jones K, 1987: Lead nephropathy: In-vivo X-ray fluorescence (XRF) for assessing body lead stores, in In-vivo body composition studies. Ellis KJ, Yasumura SY, Morgen W (eds). The Institute of Physical Sciences in Medicine, London, pp. 357–362.

17. Morgan WD, Ryde SJS, Jones SJ, Wyatt RM, Hainsworth IR, Cobbold S, Evans CJ, Braithwaite RA, 1989: In-vivo measurements of cadmium and lead in occupationally-exposed workers and in an urban population. Biol Trace Elem Res 15: 1–14.

18. Skerfving S, Christoffersson J-O, Schutz A, Welinder H, Spang G, Ahlgren L, Mattson S, 1983: Biological monitoring, by in-vivo XRF measurements, of occupational exposure to lead, cadmium and mercuryhypertension with renal impairment. N Engl J Med 309: 17–21.

19. Van de Vyver FL, D'Haese PC, Visser WJ, Elsiviers MM, Knippenberg LJ, Lamberts LV, Wedeen RP, DeBroe ME, 1988: Bone lead in dialysis patients. Kidney Int 33: 601–7.

20. Cory-Shlecta D, Weiss B, Cox C, 1987: Mobilization and redistribution of lead over the course of calcium disodium ethylenediamine tetra-acetic acid chelation therapy. J. Pharm Exptl Ther 243: 804–13.

21. Fowler B, Silbergeld E (eds), 19xx: Proc int symposium on lead in bone, environ health perspect (in press).

22. Rosen JF, Markowitz ME, Bijur PE, Jenks ST, Weilopolski L, Kalef-Ezra JA, Slatkin DN, 1989: L-line X-ray fluorescence of cortical bone lead compared with CaNa$_2$EDTA test in lead-toxic children: Public health implications, Proc Nat Acad Sci USA 86: 685–9.

23. Schidlovsky G, Jones K, Burger DE, Milder FL, Hu H, 19XX: Distribution of lead in human bone: II. Proton microprobe measurements. Proc int symposium on in vivo body

composition studies, 20–23 June 1989, Plenum Press, Toronto (In press).

24. Wedeen RP, 1985: Blood lead levels, dietary calcium, and hypertension. Ann Int Med 102: 403–4.

25. Batuman V, Landy E, Maesaka JK, Wedeen RP, 1983: Contribution of lead to hypertension with renal impairment. N Engl J Med 309: 17–21.

Prevention of bone disease in renal failure

HARTMUT H. MALLUCHE, MARIE-CLAUDE FAUGERE &
LAURENCE R.I. BAKER

Histologic evidence of bone disease is present early in the evolution of chronic renal failure. Prevention of bone disease and hyperparathyroidism with vitamin D metabolites appears logical, but the few prospective, placebo controlled studies published involved patients with end stage renal failure [1]. Consequently, our double-blind study followed patients with mild to moderate renal impairment in an attempt to determine whether a beneficial effect upon serum biochemistry and histological abnormalities can be obtained without deleterious effects on renal function.

Sixteen of 30 patients who met inclusion criteria agreed to take part in a study of 12 months duration. Three patients were subsequently withdrawn from the study.

Initial assessment included measurement of 24-hour urinary calcium and phosphorus excretions before commencement of the study to establish baseline biochemistry. X-rays of hands, feet, clavicles and skull were made. After administration of tetracycline double label over a twenty-day period, an initial bone biopsy of the iliac crest was used to profile baseline histomorphometric parameters.

Patients were asymptomatic with normal serum alkaline phosphatase concentrations and bone radiographs. All subjects had woven osteoid and elevated numbers of bone resorbing and forming cells, findings that can be ascribed to increased PTH activity on bone. Seven individuals had elevated PTH levels; seven had low serum $1,25(OH)_2D$.

Patients were randomly allocated to receive $1,25(OH)_2D_3$ or placebo. The initial dose of 0.25 μg daily was doubled to 0.5 μg between 4 and 8 weeks after commencement of treatment. This proved to be a too high dose in most patients. Hypercalcemia or hypercalciuria occurred. This finding was associated with a rise in urinary calcium excretion, increased serum creatinine levels and a fall in creatinine clearance and indicates that fre-

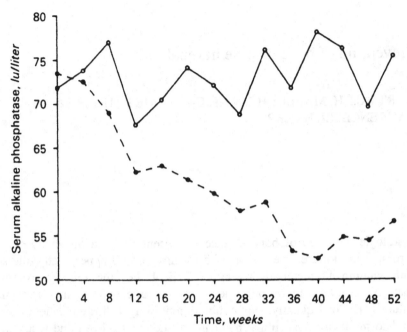

Figure 1. Serum alkaline phosphatase during 52 weeks of administration of 1,25(OH)$_2$D$_3$ or placebo to patients with moderate renal failure. Symbols are: (O---O) placebo; (Å---Å) 1,25(OH)$_2$D$_3$. (Reproduced, with permission, from LRI Baker *et al.* Kidney International 35: 661–9, 1989.)

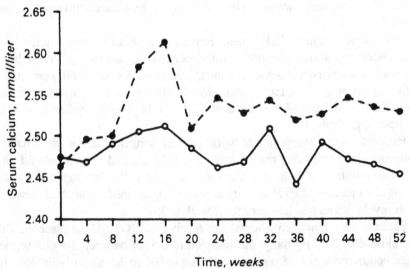

Figure 2. Serum calcium during 52 weeks of administration of 1,25(OH)$_2$D$_3$ or placebo to patients with moderate renal failure. Symbols are: (O---O) placebo; (Å---Å) 1,25(OH)$_2$D$_3$. (Reproduced, with permission, from LRI Baker *et al.* Kidney International 35: 661–9, 1989.)

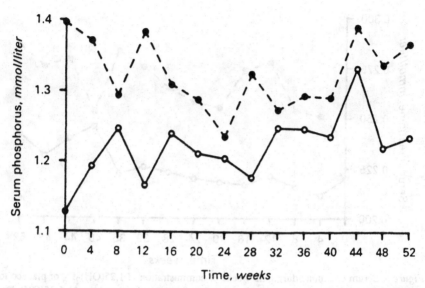

Figure 3. Serum phosphorus during 52 weeks of administration of 1,25(OH)₂D₃ or placebo to patients with moderate renal failure. Symbols are: (O---O) placebo; (Å---Å) 1,25(OH)₂D₃. (Reproduced, with permission, from LRI Baker *et al.* Kidney International 35: 661–9, 1989.)

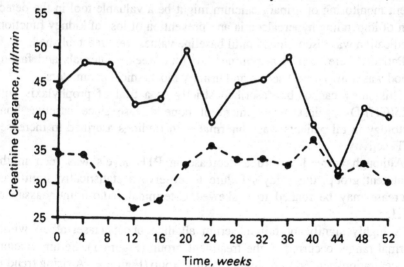

Figure 4. Creatinine clearance during 52 weeks of administration of 1,25(OH)₂D₃ or placebo to patients with moderate renal failure. Symbols are: (O---O) placebo; (Å---Å) 1,25(OH)₂D₃. (Reproduced, with permission, from LRI Baker *et al.* Kidney International 35: 661–9, 1989.)

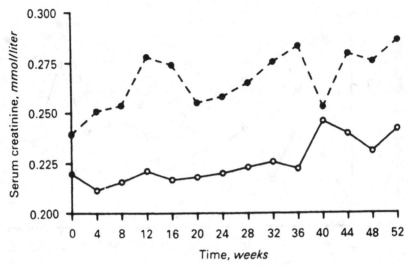

Figure 5. Serum creatinine during 52 weeks of administration of 1,25(OH)$_2$D$_3$ or placebo to patients with moderate renal failure. Symbols are: (O---O) placebo; (À---À) 1,25(OH)$_2$D$_3$. (Reproduced, with permission, from LRI Baker *et al.* Kidney International 35: 661–9, 1989.)

quent monitoring of urinary calcium might be a valuable tool in the detection of impending hypercalcemia and prevention of loss of kidney function. Medication was discontinued until baseline values were reestablished.

Patients were seen at a minimum of four weekly intervals and fasting blood was drawn for all serum and urinary biochemical parameters.

This study cannot be described strictly as a trial of prophylaxis with 1,25(OH)$_2$D$_3$ against development of bone disease since baseline bone histology in all patients was abnormal with findings ascribed to increased PTH activity.

Although a trend toward a decrease in PTH levels was seen in the treatment group, the study's failure to observe a statistically significant decrease may be related to a skewed C-terminal radio-immunoassay of PTH.

A highly significant fall in serum alkaline phosphatase, albeit within normal range, occurred in the treatment group (Figure 1). Serum calcium concentrations tended to be higher in this group (Figure 2). A rising trend in serum phosphorus (Figure 3) occurred in the control group, but not in the treatment group, the difference being statistically significant.

Urinary phosphorus was within the normal range in both groups throughout the study. Urinary calcium excretion did not differ significantly throughout.

The study provides histologic evidence for the amelioration of hyperparathyroid changes. Further deterioration of mineralization was not observed in the treatment group, and bone turnover was decreased. However, decreased bone turnover is desirable only to the degree that elevated turnover is brought back to normal. Low or below normal levels must be avoided. Further studies are needed to determine whether smaller doses of $1,25(OH)_2D_3$ or intermittent therapy may avoid suppression of bone turnover.

During the course of the study, there was no significant deterioration of renal function attributable to treatment with $1,25(OH)_2D_3$ (Figures 4–5). This experience contrasts with that of two other studies conducted in 1978 [2] and 1980 [3]. In those studies, dosages of $1,25(OH)_2D_3$ given were much larger, patients selected suffered from end-stage renal failure and assessment of serum and urinary biochemistries was less stringent.

The long-term goals of $1,25(OH)_2D_3$ treatment in patients with mild to moderate renal impairment is to protect bones from the consequences of progressive renal failure and to prevent parathyroid hyperplasia thereby obviating the need for new surgery. Our study shows that those goals are in part realizable.

Observation of much larger numbers of patients over a longer period of time is required to determine whether the need for neck exploration can be reduced by $1,25(OH)_2D_3$ administration.

Long-term $1,25(OH)_2D_3$ administration in patients should be carried out only if frequent and meticulous follow-up can be ensured (monitoring of urine and serum calcium and renal function), and lower doses than those used in end-stage renal failure are prescribed.

References

1. Baker LRI, Muir JW, Sharman VL, Abrams SML, Greenwood RN, Cattel WR, Goodwin FJ, Marsh FP, Adami S, Hately W, Hattersley LA, Morgan AG, Papapoulos SE, Revell PA, Tucker AK, Chaput de Saintonge DM, O'Riordan JLH, 1986: Controlled trial of calcitriol in haemodialysis patients. Clin Nephrol 26: 185–91.
2. Christiansen C, Rodbro P, Christiansen MS, Hartnack B, Transbol I, 1978: Deterioration of renal function during treatment of chronic renal failure with 1,25-dihydroxycholecalciferol. Lancet ii: 700–3.
3. Healy MD, Malluche HM, Goldstein DA, Singer FR, Massry ST, 1980: Effects of long-term therapy with calcitriol in patients with moderate renal failure. Arch Intern Med 14: 1030–3.

Kidney function, hypertension and clinical diabetic nephropathy in type 1 diabetes

JENS SANDAHL CHRISTIANSEN

Introduction

The complications of insulin-dependent diabetes mellitus (IDDM) leading to the clinical syndromes of diabetic retinopathy, diabetic nephropathy, diabetic cardiomyopathy, and diabetic neuropathy are well known. The consequence of these manifestations, the late diabetic syndrome, is also well recognized. Diabetic nephropathy is probably the most serious complication and it is, therefore, not surprising that an increasing and continuous interest in the diabetic kidney has been seen during the last two decades. Much work has been done studying the morphological consequences of diabetes on the kidney, e.g. the classical work by Østerby et al. [1], the experimental studies by Rasch [2], as well as the abundance of information coming from the Minneapolis groups [3]. The functional changes in the diabetic kidney have been comprehensively studied by Mogensen [4] and others with increasing interest, since recent studies have pointed towards a possible causal relationship between the early functional alterations and the development of clinical diabetic nephropathy [5, 6]. This review deals with our present knowledge of the epidemiology of diabetic nephropathy, the early haemodynamic disturbances, and the development of hypertension.

Epidemiology

Clinical diabetic nephropathy, i.e. persistent proteinuria, is the most severe clinical manifestation of microangiopathy in patients with insulin-dependent diabetes mellitus. Detailed epidemiological studies in IDDM have shown that, although the last decades have seen an increase in life expec-

M. E. De Broe and G. A. Verpooten (eds.): Prevention in Nephrology, 79–87.
© 1991 Kluwer Academic Publishers. Printed in the Netherlands.

80

tancy for these patients, they still have a significantly higher mortality rate than the general background population [7].

The dominating factor leading to the reduced life expectancy of IDDM patients is the development of diabetic renal disease as diagnosed by the presence of persistent proteinuria. Patients with persistent normal urinary albumin excretion have a low relative mortality and, indeed, a near normal life expectancy, whereas the median life expectancy after the onset of persistent proteinuria is only 6–7 years [8] (Figure 1). The latter figures, however, do not take into account the possible impact of intensive treatment, i.e. aggressive treatment of hypertension, dialyses, and renal transplantation.

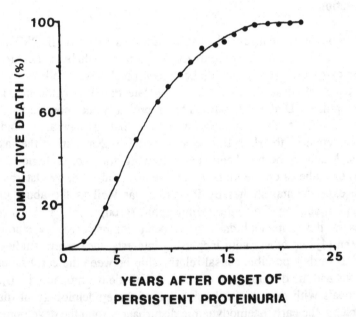

Figure 1. Cumulative death rate in IDDM patients after the onset of persistent proteinuria [9]. (Reprinted with permission, © 1983 Springer-Verlag, Heidelberg, Berlin.)

It has been demonstrated that the cumulative incidence of diabetic nephropathy in IDDM is as high as 40–50% [9]. Thus, more than half of the patients seem to escape from this severe complication. This finding has lead to speculations that only a fraction of the patients are indeed susceptible to development of proteinuria and several genetic factors have been suggested as factors involving increased susceptibility [10]. On the other hand, more recent studies have demonstrated a tendency towards a decrease in prevalence and incidence of proteinuria in IDDM in the last decade [11, 12], suggesting environmental and metabolic factors to be important for the development of this complication.

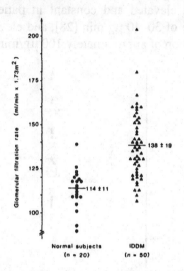

Figure 2. Glomerular filtration rate in young normoalbuminuric IDDM patients as compared to normal subjects.

Increased urinary albumin excretion has also been shown to be associated with a decrease in the survival rate in non-insulin dependent diabetics [13].

Haemodynamics

Numerous studies of GFR have been carried out since the early suggestion by Cambier [14] and Spühler [15] that GFR might be above normal level in a number of diabetic patients. At the onset of IDDM, GFR is increased by more than 40% [4, 16]. Initial insulin treatment is followed by reduction but not complete correction of the hyperfiltration [4, 16] and during conditions of ordinary metabolic control on standard insulin injection therapy, GFR has consistently been reported to be elevated by 20–25% in non-proteinuric diabetic children and adults after 1–15 years of diabetes duration [17–26] (Figure 2). Also in patients with long-standing diabetes still without proteinuria, GFR is usually increased [27, 28]. However, approximately

82

half of IDDM patients develop persistent proteinuria within 40 years of onset; increased urinary albumin excretion signals a steady decline in GFR [28, 29]. In the interphase between normal albumin excretion and clinical proteinuria, i.e. at the stage of incipient nephropathy or 'microalbuminuria', GFR has been found elevated and constant in patients with an urinary albumin excretion rate of 30–40 µg/min [28], and elevated but declining in patients with an excretion of approximately 100 µg/min [30].

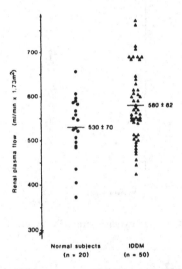

Figure 3. Renal plasma flow in young normoalbuminuric IDDM patients as compared to normal subjects.

An increased kidney size in patients having IDDM was originally described by Mogensen and Andersen [20] and later confirmed by others [22, 24, 25]. Kidney size is also increased at diagnosis [16, 31]. It has been proposed that the increased kidney size is the main cause of the elevated GFR in IDDM [4, 20], a suggestion supported by the finding of a covaria-tion in GFR and kidney size measured before and after three months of initial insulin therapy in newly diagnosed patients [31]. That concept, however, has been seriously challenged, since a dichotomy between renal size and glomerular function has been demonstrated [16]. Thus, initial treatment of newly diagnosed IDDM patients induced a substantial and highly significant decline in GFR before any reduction in kidney volume [16]. This finding is in accordance with a morphometric study on kidney biopsies from newly diagnosed IDDM patients in which the enlargement of the glomerular filtration surface area was found unchanged after five weeks of insulin treatment [32] – a period where a considerable decline in GFR would be expected. Thus, the increased kidney size is not a primary variable, but rather represents adaptation to the increase in function.

Renal plasma flow is also significantly elevated in short-term IDDM patients, although not to the same extent as the elevation of GFR [4, 33] (Figure 3). The glomerular filtration rate has also been found to be significantly elevated in experimental diabetic animal models [34, 35]. Hyperperfusion has been demonstrated in several other vascular beds in diabetics, findings that correspond well with the recent observations of increased cardiac output in short-term IDDM [36]. On the basis of these clinical and experimental studies, it has been suggested that hyperperfusion and decreased pre-capillary resistance play a role in the genesis of diabetic microangiopathy, because the effect of hyperperfusion and decreased pre-capillary resistance results in increased hydrostatic capillary pressure and extravasation of plasma proteins [6].

Antihypertensive treatment

Arterial hypertension in IDDM is closely related to the onset of clinical proteinuria [37]. Hypertension is not frequently observed early in disease and mean arterial blood pressure of newly diagnosed diabetics is not higher than the background population. It is presently highly controversial whether there is an association between blood pressure level early in disease and the subsequent development of clinical diabetic nephropathy.

A slight but significant elevation of blood pressure has been observed in patients with microalbuminuria [38]. Also in patients with overt proteinuria but with normal serum creatinine levels, blood pressure is significantly higher compared with otherwise matched patients without proteinuria [37]. Thus, it can be concluded that hypertension is a very early phenomenon in diabetic nephropathy, but it is still uncertain whether it is the increase in blood pressure that causes the process leading to microalbuminuria and, subsequently, nephropathy, or whether increased urinary albumin excretion and enhancement of blood pressure are simultaneous consequences of a series of intra- and extra-renal vascular events.

So far only one study has been able to demonstrate that it might be possible by means of improved metabolic control to influence the clinical cause of diabetic nephropathy. In a two-year prospective study in patients

84

with microalbuminuria, the Steno group demonstrated that the increase in blood pressure in IDDM patients with incipient nephropathy was arrested in a group of patients treated with continuous subcutaneous insulin infusion (insulin pumps) as compared to a control group [39].

Several studies have suggested that it is possible to reduce the intra-glomerular capillary pressure in as well normo-albuminuric as well as microalbuminuric patients by means of dietary protein restriction or treatment with antihypertensive agents. It has, for example, been shown that in normotensive normoalbuminuric IDDM patients the administration of angiotensin converting enzyme inhibitors results in a decrease in fractional albumin clearance [40] (Figure 4).

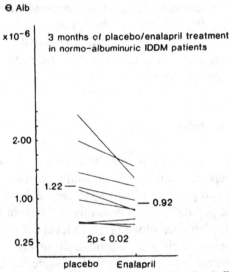

Figure 4. Fractional albumin excretion in young normoalbuminuric IDDM patients during 3 months of treatment with ACE inhibitor and placebo respectively.

In 1976, Mogensen demonstrated that short-term antihypertensive treatment of IDDM patients with diabetic nephropathy reduced urinary albumin excretion [41]. This finding led him to suggest that antihypertensive treatment might postpone renal insufficiency in diabetic nephropathy. It was subsequently demonstrated that long-term antihypertensive treatment in such patients could slow the rate of decline in the glomerular filtration rate and in this way probably postpone end-stage renal failure in IDDM patients with diabetic nephropathy [42–44]. Several studies are presently ongoing to elucidate whether antihypertensive treatment initiated early in the course of nephropathy, i.e. during the microalbuminuric stage, might have a beneficial effect upon the development and/or further progression of kidney disease in these patients.

Of particular interest is the very recent observation that the early antihypertensive treatment regimen in diabetic nephropathy is associated with a highly significant improvement of survival in these patients. Thus, Mathiesen and coworkers compared survival in two cohorts of IDDM patients followed at the same hospital. The first group developed persistent proteinuria in the time period from 1959 to 1979, while the second cohort developed persistent proteinuria in the period 1979 to 1983. In the latter cohort the 'early treatment' regimen had been used. It was demonstrated that when early antihypertensive treatment was given to patients with nephropathy, the percentage who survived for more than 8 years has increased from 48% to 87% [45].

Similar results have also been reported by Parving [46]. Thus, it can be concluded that the prognosis of diabetic nephropathy has improved during the past decades – most probably due to effective antihypertensive therapy.

References

1. Østerby R, 1975: Early phases in the development of diabetic glomerulopathy. A quantitative electron microscopic study. Acta Med Scand 197: suppl. 574: 3–82.
2. Rasch R, 1980: Prevention of diabetic glomerulopathy by insulin treatment. An experimental study. Thesis. Aarhus.
3. Mauer SM, Steffes MW, Ellis EN, Sutherland DER, Brown DM, Goetz FC, 1984: Structural-functional relationships in diabetic nephropathy. J Clin Invest 74: 1143–55.
4. Mogensen CE, 1972: Kidney function and glomerular permeability to macromolecules in juvenile diabetes. Dan Med Bull suppl. 19: 1–40.
5. Hostetter TH, Rennke GH, Brenner BM, 1982: The case for intrarenal hypertension in the initiation and progression of diabetic and other glomerulopathies. Am J Med 72: 375–80.
6. Parving H-H, Viberti GC, Keen H, Christiansen JS, Lassen NA, 1983: The hemodynamic origin of diabetic microangiopathy. Metabolism 32: 943–9.
7. Green A, Borch-Johnsen K, Andersen PK, Hougaard P, Keiding N, Kreiner S, Deckert T, 1985: Relative mortality of Type 1 (insulin-dependent) diabetes in Denmark: 1933–1981. Diabetologia 28: 339–42.
8. Andersen AR, Andersen JK, Christiansen JS, Deckert T, 1978: Prognosis for juvenile diabetics with nephropathy and failing renal function. Acta Med Scand 203: 131–4.
9. Andersen AR, Christiansen JS, Andersen JK, Kreiner S, Deckert T, 1983: Diabetic nephropathy in type 1 (insulin-dependent) diabetes: An epidemiological study. Diabetologia 25: 496–501.
10. Barbosa J, Saner B, 1984: Do genetic factors play a role in the pathogenesis of diabetic

microangiopathy? Diabetologia 27: 487–92.

11. Kofoed-Enevoldsen A, Borch-Johnsen K, Kreiner S, Nerup J, Deckert T, 1987: Declining incidence of persistent proteinuria in Type 1 (insulin-dependent) diabetic patients in Denmark. Diabetes 36: 205–9.

12. Krolewski AS, Warram JH, Christlieb AR, Buscik EJ, Kahn CR, 1985: The changing natural history of nephropathy in Type 1 diabetes. Am J Med 78: 785–94.

13. Schmitz A, Vaeth M, 1988: Microalbuminuria: Major risk factor in non-insulin-dependent diabetes – A 10-year follow-up study of 503 patients. Diab Med 5: 126–34.

14. Cambier P, 1934: Application de la théorie de Rehberg à l'étude clinique des affections rénales et du diabète. Ann Méd 35: 273–299.

15. Spühler O, 1946: Zur Physio-pathologie der Niere. Huber, Bern, pp. 45–9.

16. Christiansen JS, Gammelgaard J, Tronier B, Svendsen PA, Parving H-H, 1982: Kidney function and size in diabetics, before and during initial insulin treatment. Kidney Int 21: 683–8.

17. Stalder G, Schmid R, 1959: Severe functional disorders of glomerular capillaries and renal hemodynamics in treated diabetes mellitus during childhood. Ann Paediat 193: 129–38.

18. Ditzel J, Schwartz M, 1967: Abnormally increased glomerular filtration rate in short-term insulin-treated diabetic subjects. Diabetes 16: 264–7.

19. Ditzel J, Junker K, 1972: Abnormal glomerular filtration rate, renal plasma flow, and renal protein excretion in recent and short-term diabetics. Br Med J 2: 13–19.

20. Mogensen CE, Andersen MJF, 1973: Increased kidney size and glomerular filtration rate in early juvenile diabetes. Diabetes 22: 706–13.

21. Parving H-H, Nier I, Deckert T, Evrin P-E, Nielsen SL, Lyngsøe J, Mogensen CE, Rørth M, Svendsen PAA, Trap-Jensen J, Lassen, 1976: The effect of metabolic regulation on microvascular permeability to small and large molecules in short-term juvenile diabetics. Diabetologia 12: 161–6.

22. Madácsy L, Kiss S, Borsodi A, 1978: The size of the kidneys of diabetic children in the early stage of the disease. Orvosi Hetilab 119: 317–20.

23. Brøchner-Mortensen J, Ditzel J, Mogensen CE, Rødbro P, 1979: Microvascular permeability to albumin and glomerular filtration rate in diabetic and normal children. Diabetologia 16: 307–11.

24. Christiansen JS, Gammelgaard J, Frandsen M, Parving H-H, 1981: Increased kidney size, glomerular filtration rate and renal plasma flow in short-term insulin-dependent diabetics. Diabetologia 20: 451–6.

25. Puig JG, Antón FM, Grande C, Pallardo LF, Arnalich F, Gil A, Vázquez JJ, García AM, 1981: Relation of kidney size to kidney function in early insulin-dependent diabetes. Diabetologia 21: 363–7.

26. Nyberg G, Granerus G, Aurell M, 1982: Renal extraction ratios for 51 Cr-EDTA, PAH, and glucose in early insulin-dependent diabetic patients. Kidney Int 21: 706–8.

27. Mogensen CE, 1971: Glomerular filtration rate and renal plasma flow in short-term and long-term juvenile diabetes mellitus. Scand J Clin Lab Invest 28: 91–100.

28. Mogensen CE, 1976: Progression of nephropathy in long-term diabetics with proteinuria and effect of initial antihypertensive treatment. Scand J Clin Lab Invest 36: 383–8.

29. Parving H-H, Smidt UM, Friisberg B, Bonnevie-Nielsen V, Andersen AR, 1981: A

prospective study of glomerular filtration rate and arterial blood pressure in insulin-dependent diabetes with diabetic nephropathy. Diabetologia 20: 457–61.

30. Bending JJ, Viberti GC, Redmund S, Watkins J, Keen H, 1984: Intermittent clinical proteinuria and renal function in diabetes: Evolution and the effect of glycemic control (abstract). Diabetologia 27: 255A–6A.

31. Mogensen CE, Andersen MJF, 1975: Increased kidney size and glomerular filtration rate in untreated juvenile diabetics: Normalization by insulin-treatment. Diabetologia 11: 221–4.

32. Kroustrup JP, Gundersen HJG, Østerby R, 1977: Glomerular size and structure in diabetes mellitus. III. Early enlargement of the capillary surface. Diabetologia 13: 207–10.

33. Christiansen JS, 1984: On the pathogenesis of the increased glomerular filtration rate in short-term insulin-dependent diabetes. Dan Med Bull 31: 349–61.

34. Hostetter TH, Troy TL, Brenner BM, 1981: Glomerular hemodynamics in experimental diabetes mellitus. Kidney Int 19: 410–15.

35. Jensen PK, Christiansen JS, Steven K, Parving H-H, 1981: Renal function in strep-tozotocin diabetic rats. Diabetologia 21: 409–14.

36. Thuesen L, Christiansen JS, Mogensen CE, Henningsen P, 1988: Cardiac hyperfunction in insulin dependent diabetic patients developing microvascular complications. Diabetes 37: 851–6.

37. Parving H-H, Andersen AR, Smidt UM, Oxenbøll B, Edsberg B, Christiansen JS, 1983: Diabetic nephropathy and arterial hypertension. Diabetologia 24: 10–12.

38. Mathiesen ER, Oxenbøll B, Johansen K, Svendsen PAA, Deckert T, 1984: Incipient diabetic nephropathy in type 1 (insulin-dependent) diabetes. Diabetologia 26: 406–10.

39. Feldt-Rasmussen B, Mathiesen ER, Deckert T, 1986: Effect of two years of strict metabolic control on progression of incipient nephropathy in insulin-dependent diabetes. Lancet ii: 1300–4.

40. Pedersen MM, Schmitz A, Pedersen EB, Danielsen H, Christiansen JS, 1988: Acute and long-term renal effects of angiotensin converting enzyme inhibition in normotensive, normoalbuminuric insulin-dependent diabetics. Diabetic Medicine 5: 562–9.

41. Mogensen CE, 1976: Progression of nephropathy in long-term diabetics with proteinuria and effect of initial anti-hypertensive treatment. Scand J Clin Lab Invest 36: 383–8.

42. Mogensen CE, 1982: Long-term antihypertensive treatment inhibiting progression of diabetic nephropathy. Br Med J 285: 685–8.

43. Parving H-H, Andersen AR, Smidt UM, Svendsen PA, 1983: Early aggressive antihypertensive treatment reduce rate of decline in kidney function in diabetic nephropathy. Lancet i: 1175–9.

44. Parving H-H, Hommel E, Nielsen MD, Giese J, 1989: Effect of captopril on blood pressure and kidney function in normotensive insulin dependent diabetics with nephropathy. Br Med J 299: 533–6.

45. Mathiesen EM, Borch-Johnsen K, Jensen DV, Deckert T, 1989: Antihypertensive treatment improves survival in patients with Type 1 (insulin-dependent) diabetes and nephropathy (abstract). Diabetologia 32: 515A.

46. Parving H-H, Hommel E, 1989: Prognosis in diabetic nephropathy. Br Med J 299: 230–3.

Drug management of hyperlipemia

J.P. DESLYPERE

Coronary heart disease (CHD) is a major cause of death in most industrialized countries, and is the leading killer in North America, exacting an enormous personal and public toll. Numerous studies have produced a growing body of irrefutable evidence that dyslipidemias, in particular elevated levels of total cholesterol and low density lipoprotein (LDL) cholesterol, are major contributors to atherosclerosis – the buildup of fatty deposits (plaque) that eventually clog arteries and directly cause about 85% of all cardiovascular mortality. More importantly, investigators have confirmed that reducing total and LDL cholesterol in conjunction with raising high density lipoprotein (HDL) cholesterol lowers the incidence of CHD and its devastating effects, especially myocardial infarction. While the evidence is compelling, many clinicians are still uncertain of the role that lipids and lipoproteins play in CHD and why they should be treated.

Why treat? (Table 1)

International research over the past several decades has yielded a wealth of data about the relationship of lipid disorders to coronary disease. In response, the medical consensus has shifted markedly in favor of more aggressive therapy to lower elevated lipids, for the general population and especially for those at high risk of cardiovascular disease. The direct link between high plasma cholesterol and CHD is based on:

- the naturally occurring development of atherosclerosis in animals and humans,
- genetic studies showing early, severe occurrence of CHD in patients with familial hypercholesterolemia and no other coronary risk factors,

M. E. De Broe and G. A. Verpooten (eds.): Prevention in Nephrology, 89–105.
© 1991 *Kluwer Academic Publishers. Printed in the Netherlands.*

- animal experiments in which atherosclerosis can be produced only by inducing high cholesterol levels,
- epidemiological studies linking high-fat diets and increased blood cholesterol to CHD. Prospective epidemiological studies, most notably the Framingham Heart Study [1] and the PROCAM study [2], have demonstrated that total serum cholesterol and CHD incidence are directly related and that HDL cholesterol is inversely proportional to CHD. (This association is strongest in middle-aged men and less pronounced in older persons. A similar but delayed pattern of risk and treatment benefits is presumed, but not proven, to exist for women, whose rates of CHD become similar to those of men in the decades after menopause.) When blood cholesterol measures above 240 mg/dl, the rate of CHD is twice that found with cholesterol levels of 200 mg/dl.

Table 1. Reduction of total cholesterol by drugs: Major clinical trials

Trial	N	Duration (years)	Drug used	Average TC change (%)	CHD change (%)
Coronary Drug Project	8,341	4.5	Niacin	−10	−27 Nonfatal MI
LRC-CPPT	3,806	7.4	Cholestyramine	−8.5	−19 Nonfatal MI −24 CHD deaths
WHO	15,754	5	Clofibrate	−9	−20 Nonfatal MI
Helsinki Heart Study	4,081	5	Gemfibrozil	−11	−34 CHD (fatal, non-fatal MI; cardiac death)

N = number of patients; TC = total cholesterol; CHD = coronary heart disease; MI = myocardial infarction.

Clinical studies have demonstrated that lowering elevated cholesterol *reduces* CHD risk. Landmark investigations include:
- The LRC-CPPT (Lipid Research Clinics-Coronary Primary Prevention Trial [3, 4]). This double-blind study, completed in 1983 by the United States' National Heart, Lung, and Blood Institute compared the effects of a low-fat diet plus the cholesterol-lowering drug cholestyramine with those of diet therapy alone in about 3800 middle-aged men. Over a seven-year period, the drug-treated group experienced a 19% lower

incidence of CHD. The study found that for every 1% reduction in total cholesterol, there was a 2% decrease in heart attack incidence.
- CLAS (Cholesterol-Lowering Atherosclerosis Study [5]). Treatment with both diet and drugs (colestipol and nicotinic acid) produced not only a significant slowdown in the *rate* of atherosclerosis, but also evidence of regression of atherosclerotic lesions in 16% of patients treated vs. 2% in the placebo group. This effect was demonstrated angiographically in patients who had undergone coronary artery bypass grafting. The study participants on drug therapy showed a 26% decrease in total cholesterol and a 43% decrease in LDL cholesterol. There was also a 37% elevation in HDL cholesterol in patients given the drug.
- The Helsinki Heart Study [6, 7]. Published in 1987, this study provided the first strong clinical evidence that increasing HDL with drug treatment added an additional reduction in CHD beyond that obtained by lowering LDL and total cholesterol. This double-blind, randomized trial compared fatal and non-fatal heart attacks in 4081 men with high blood cholesterol and no apparent CHD. All followed low-fat diets, but approximately one-half were also treated with gemfibrozil, while the other group received placebo. The drug-treated group had a 34% lower rate of CHD. Over a five-year period, the drug treatment group had an average 8% decrease in LDL, 8% decrease in total cholesterol and an average 10% increase in HDL.

These clinical trials reinforce the benefits to be gained by controlling dyslipidemias. And, since the first symptom of CHD is often the last (sudden death), identification of hyperlipidemic patients serves both a prognostic and therapeutic purpose. Here, the primary care physician plays a vital role and is assisted by the current surge of reporting on cholesterol that has raised public awareness and concern. There has never been a better time to screen patients for lipid disorders, nor a better reason to do so.

Whom to treat

The diagnosis and management of lipid disorders is complex and challenging, requiring cooperation among the physician, patient and other members of the health care team. Treatment decisions must be based on direct lipid measurements and on a complete cardiovascular risk profile.

In the United States, the federal government has launched the National

Cholesterol Education Program (NCEP) [8], an intensive campaign to alert physicians and patients to the importance of treating lipid disorders. According to the NCEP guidelines up to 50% of people in most Western nations may be at increased risk for heart attack due to elevated blood lipids (defined as total cholesterol above 200 mg/dl). In Europe, a 1988 Policy Statement of the European Atherosclerosis Society defined the same cholesterol level as a risk cutpoint [9].

In simplified terms, the main categories of lipid disorders that increase CHD risk include:

- *Hypercholesterolemia*: an abnormally high level of cholesterol in the blood. Many experts now consider desirable serum cholesterol levels to be below 200 mg/dl, LDL cholesterol to be below 130 mg/dl, and HDL to be above 35 mg/dl. It has also been suggested that an ideal total cholesterol to HDL ratio is less than 4, and an ideal LDL to HDL ratio is less than 3. (The NCEP guidelines stop short of recommending such ratios as a basis for treatment.)
- *Hypertriglyceridemia*: elevated levels of triglycerides (defined by an NIH Consensus Panel as above 500 mg/dl). Normal triglycerides, which vary with meals, range from 50 mg/dl to 250 mg/dl; in the fasting state, they should be less than 200 mg/dl. While hypertriglyceridemia does not appear to be an independent risk for CHD, it is often associated with low levels of HDL. Importantly, obesity, diabetes, excess alcohol use, or certain drugs (including estrogen and beta blockers) may raise triglyceride and lower HDL cholesterol. Triglyceride levels above 1000 mg/dl require urgent treatment to prevent pancreatitis; moderate hypertriglyceridemia usually responds to restriction of fat and calories and weight loss.
- *Mixed dyslipidemia*: a concurrent excess of cholesterol and triglycerides. This presents a more complicated therapeutic picture than either condition alone.
- *Hypoalphalipoproteinemia*, or low levels of HDL (below 35 mg/dl). Exercising, stopping smoking, and losing weight all may help elevate protective HDL cholesterol; some triglyceride-lowering drugs may also elevate HDL cholesterol.

Ideally, every patient should have total blood cholesterol levels measured by age 20 and rechecked at intervals throughout life as needed (at least once every five years). Total cholesterol, measured on two separate visits in a

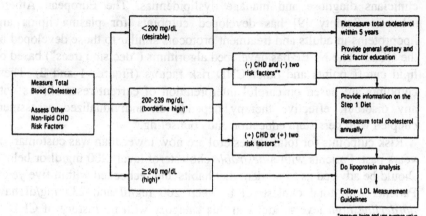

Fig. 1.

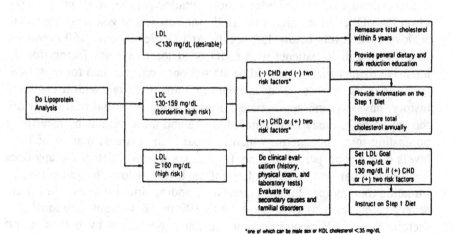

Fig. 2.

nonfasting patient, provides a convenient, cost-effective first step in lipid evaluation.

Both the United States and Europe have established guidelines to help clinicians diagnose and manage dyslipidemias. The European Athero-sclerosis Society [9] has developed cutpoints for plasma lipids and lipoproteins in adults and treatment protocols similar to those developed by the NCEP. The NCEP has developed algorithms ("decision trees") based on lipid cutoff points and other CHD risk factors (Figures 1 and 2). These cutpoints are based on careful interpretation of current research. As with any disorder, effective therapy depends on individualized assessment coupled with persistent education and counseling.

Risk cutpoints for total cholesterol are now lower than was customary in years past. Patients with a *desirable* cholesterol level (200 mg/dl or below) should be advised as to prudent diet habits and rechecked within five years. Patients with total cholesterol between 200 mg/dl and 239 mg/dl have *borderline high* levels; adults in this category with no history of CHD or CHD factors should receive information on the Step One diet and be retested annually. Adults in this range who have two or more other cardiac risk factors (one of which may be male sex), or those whose total choles-terol is 240 mg/dl or greater with or without other risks are at *high risk* and should have further lipoprotein analysis, with an examination of LDL, HDL and triglyceride levels.

Lipoprotein analysis provides a more detailed picture of actual risk. The lower the LDL, and the higher the HDL, the better. The goal of therapy is to achieve LDL levels below 130 mg/dl. At LDL levels over 160 mg/dl (or over 130 mg/dl in patients with CHD or at least two risk factors for it), intensive dietary therapy should be started once other causes for high LDL (such as other diseases or drug treatment) are ruled out with a complete history, physical, and appropriate testing. During an initial trial of dietary therapy, progress may be monitored at one and three months by measuring nonfasting total cholesterol, which is usually an adequate marker of LDL levels over a short period of time. If, after six months, dietary therapy does not lower total and LDL cholesterol to levels below the cutpoints for initiating therapy (see Figure 1), consider adding drug treatment. In certain severe cases, such as LDL levels over 190 mg/dl without additional risk factors, the NCEP recommends immediate intervention by both diet and drug therapy.

The presence of additional risk factors makes dietary or drug intervention even more important in controlling dyslipidemias and preventing CHD.

Smoking and hypertension are two other risk factors that demand equally intensive efforts at control. Other relevant conditions include HDL cholesterol levels below 35 mg/dl, obesity, sedentary lifestyle, diabetes, family history of premature CHD (heart attack in immediate family member before age 55), or history of coronary events. Patients must participate actively in controlling these risks.

How to treat

Diet is the cornerstone of therapy for dyslipidemias. For many patients, weight control and reducing dietary fat and cholesterol are sufficient to lower total and LDL cholesterol to acceptable levels. Pessimism about patient's compliance should not deter adequate efforts at modifying diet; food advertising reflects a widespread consumer demand for information related to "heart-healthy" eating. Patients need solid information and strong encouragement.

Dietary intervention does require intensive, time-consuming and knowledgeable counseling.

The basic dietary modifications for the Step One diet, as defined by the American Heart Association and endorsed by the NCEP, consist of keeping fat intake to no more than 30% of total calories, and saturated fats to no more than 10% of total calories. In addition, dietary cholesterol should be limited to no more than 300 mg per day (about the amount in one egg yolk). These goals can be reached through moderate restriction of fatty meats, organ meats, egg yolks, fried foods, creamy or oily dressings and sauces, nonskim dairy products and commercial baked goods. To replace these fat calories, patients should be advised to choose fish, skinless poultry, skim or lowfat dairy products, and complex carbohydrates (fruits, vegetables, legumes, rice, potatoes, pasta). Low-fat cooking methods (boiling, steaming, baking or grilling) should be advocated. If diet is adhered to, and cholesterol is still too high, the Step Two diet should be prescribed, keeping fat calories to 20% of the total and saturated fat intake to 7%. The advice of a dietician is needed when progressing to the Step Two diet.

If these diet modifications fail to lower total and LDL cholesterol to levels below the cutpoint for initiating dietary therapy (see Figure 1), the addition of drug therapy may be necessary (see Table 2). Drugs, however, are not a replacement for diet; lower-fat eating habits must be continued for drug therapy to be most effective. And, since drug treatment is likely to continue for a lifetime, it should not be undertaken lightly.

Table 2. Lipid-lowering drugs: Dosages, actions, and side effects

Drug	Dosage	Mechanisms of action	Effects on lipid and lipoprotein metabolism	Major side effects
Bile acid sequestrants				
Cholestyramine	8–12 g bid	Binds intestinal bile	⇓ LDL (major)	GI distress Constipation Interference with absorption of other drugs
Colestipol	10–15 g bid	⇑ LDL receptors	⇑ HDL (minor)	⇑ Triglycerides
HMG-CoA reductase inhibitors				
Lovastatin	20–40 mg bid	Inhibits cholesterol synthesis	⇓ LDL (major)	GI distress Insomnia ⇑ Serum transaminases ⇑ Creatine kinase
Simvastatin	10–20 mg bid	⇑ LDL receptors	⇑ HDL (minor)	

Drug	Dose	Mechanism of action	Effect on lipoproteins	Side effects
Nicotinic acid (Niacin)	0.5–1.5 g tid initiate therapy at low doses, eg. 50 mg tid and increase slowly	Inhibits secretion of lipoproteins	⇓ Triglycerides ⇓ LDL (except in some hypertriglyceridemic patients) ⇑ HDL	Flushing Itching skin/rash GI distress Hepatic dysfunction Worsening of glucose tolerance Hyperuricemia
Fibric acids Clofibrate	1 g bid	⇑ Activity of lipoprotein lipase (major)	⇓ Triglycerides	GI distress Gallstones
Gemfibrozil	600 mg bid	⇑ Intravascular breakdown of VLDL	⇑ LDL (in normo-triglyceridemic patients) ⇑ HDL	Hepatic dysfunction (mild)
Fenofibrate	100 mg tid	Inhibits cholesterol synthesis (minor)	⇓ LDL ⇑ HDL	Myopathy ⇑ Creatine (especially in renal failure) Polyuria
Probucol	500 mg bid	Enhances LDL catabolism	⇓ LDL ⇓ HDL	GI distress Prolongation of QT interval on ECG

Table 3. Expected proportion of responders[a]

Drug	Dose (g/day)	%
Bile acid sequestrants	12	70
	16	90
	20	100
Neomycin	1.5	60
Nicotinic acid	1.5	50
	2.0	75
	3.0	90
Fibrates	1.5	50

[a] Response is defined as a sustained reduction of cholesterol or LDL cholesterol of more than 10%.

Table 4. Expected percentage of patients with poor tolerance of drug

Drug	Dose (g/day)	%
Bile acid sequestrants	12	30
	16	50
Neomycin		5
Nicotinic acid	1.5	40
	3.0	80
Fibrates		1

The choice of an agent to lower cholesterol depends on the patient's lipid profile and on the cost, safety record and side effects of each agent. Major classes of cholesterol-lowering drugs include bile acid sequestrants, fibrates, HMG CoA reductase inhibitors, niacin, and probucol. Often, a combination of several agents may be indicated to lower cholesterol adequately with a minimum of side effects.

Most of the currently approved drugs are effective (Table 3). The major difficulty, however, is that they have not been well tolerated by all patients (Table 4). Even minor side effects can pose major problems when brought about by agents that must be used for decades by asymptomatic patients. Currently established agents and some new drugs are discussed below.

Bile acid sequestrants. Cholestyramine (14 to 24 g/day) and colestipol (15 to 30 g/day) are nonabsorbable agents that bind bile acids in the intestine. More cholesterol is therefore diverted to bile acid production, resulting in reduced hepatic cholesterol content. This promotes enhanced synthesis of LDL receptors and increased rates of uptake of LDL cholesterol from the blood. However, the synthesis of HMG CoA reductase, the rate-limiting enzyme of cellular cholesterol synthesis, is also activated by reduction of hepatic cholesterol, which blunts the cholesterol-lowering effect of bile acid sequestrant therapy [10]. During treatment, the serum LDL cholesterol concentration is reduced by 20% to 25%. These agents have a slight triglyceride-elevating effect that may be significant in subjects with initially high serum triglyceride levels (type IIb phenotype). Despite the proven efficacy of bile acid sequestrants, patient compliance remains a problem. Among the carefully supervised participants of the LRC-CPPT study, only a minority took the full prescribed dose of cholestyramine, six packets daily, while a significant number used an average of only zero to one packets daily [3]. Side effects include constipation (29%), flatulence, and abdominal discomfort (9%), which may be alleviated by adding fiber to the diet or by beginning with a small dose (4 g/day for cholestyramne and 5 g/day for colestipol) increasing the dose gradually. Mild and insignificant elevations of alkaline phosphatase and transaminase levels occur occasionally. Bile acid sequestrants can interfere with the absorption of concurrently administered drugs. They also increase the hepatic secretion of VLDL and can, therefore, elevate plasma TG levels.

The use of these drugs as single agents is, therefore, not advised for individuals with marked baseline hypertriglyceridemia as they can worsen the hypertriglyceridemia and enhance the risk for pancreatitis. The concurrent use of triglyceride lowering agents can allow treatment with bile acid sequestrants in hypertriglyceridemic individuals who have higher levels of LDL cholesterol. Small increases in HDLC also occur with resins.

Nicotinic acid (niacin) [11] lowers both VLDL and LDL levels. In a dose related manner beginning at about 2.5 to 3 g/day, it can reduce LDLC levels 20 to 30% and serum TG 20–50%. HDLC are moderately elevated [12]. Modification of plasma lipid levels is less dramatic when sustained release preparations of nicotine acid are used. A recent report [13] on the post treatment follow-up of coronary Drug Project patients treated with nicotinic acid demonstrated a significant reduction in total mortality as well as in coronary heart disease. The most common side effect of nicotine acid is prostaglandin mediated cutaneous flushing which occurs in nearly all individuals treated with this drug. Pretreatment with aspirine 15 to 30 min before administration of a dose of nicotinic acid minimizes the side effects. Other side effects are peptic ulcer disease, gastritis, hepatitis, glucose intolerance, hyperuricemia, acanthosis nigricans, and atrial arrhythmias. Nicotinic acid is contra-indicated in patients with a history of peptic ulcer disease or with active liver disease. Hepatitis and gastrointestinal tract distress are much more common with sustained release preparations of nicotinic acid. Compliance is therefore much poorer with these preparations. The usual dose of nicotinic acid is 1 to 3 g three times daily. Side effects are minimized if the medication is always given with meals and if the initial dose is small (50 mg three times daily), and is increased gradually over several weeks to the full therapeutic level.

The fibric acid derivatives (clofibrate, gemfibrozil, fenofibrate, bezafibrate). They speed the non-splanchnic clearance of VLDL from plasma. They also increase the secretion of cholesterol into bile leading to greater lithogenicity of bile and greater risk of gallbladder disease. They are drugs of choice for type III hyperlipemia (increased level of IDL).

Clofibrate: The first drug of the fibrate family, clofibrate (1.5 to 2 g/day) has been used as a lipid lowering agent since 1963. However, the use of clofibrate markedly declined or was discontinued in many countries, after the publication of the results of a large prospective study [14] in which clofibrate was used for treatment of moderate hypercholesterolemia. In this study, clofibrate treatment decreased coronary heart disease events significantly but was associated with excess total mortality.

Gemfibrozil: Gemfibrozil (1.2 g/day) may act both by decreasing the products of VLDL and by increasing its clearance. In hyper TG subjects this results in 50% reduction of the serum TG levels [15]. In the Helsinki Heart Study [6, 7] treatment with gemfibrozil led to an 11% decrease in LDLC level, an 11% increase in HDLC and a 34% reduction in the primary endpoint (acute myocardial infarction, CHD death); however there was no effect on total mortality.

Other fibrates [16–18]: Experience with fenofibrate, bezafibrate and ciprofibrate is accumulating. However, until now, no large scale intervention trial has been performed with any of these fibrates.

In hypertriglyceridemic patients, fibrates can cause LDL levels to rise. This might be seen despite a decrease in total plasma cholesterol levels. Other side effects of the fibrates include nausea, abdominal pain, cholelithiasis, cholecystitis, decreased libido, weight gain, myositis, ventricular arrhythmias, and drowsiness. Readjustment of the warfarine dose is required. Since fibrates are cleared by the kidneys, the dose must be adjusted in patients with renal failure.

The *3-hydroxy-3-methylglutaryl coenzyme A reductase inhibitors* (lovastatin, pravastatin, simvastatin, and fluvastatin) are the newest and most potent drugs for lowering LDL cholesterol levels [19, 20]. By inhibiting the rate-limiting enzyme of cholesterol biosynthesis, these drugs reduce the concentration of cholesterol within the hepatocyte and lead to a compensatory increase in LDL receptor activity. Thus, the clearance of LDL from plasma is enhanced. Levels of LDL cholesterol can decrease 20 to 40% in individuals treated with lovastatin; HDL cholesterol levels can increase slightly. Lovastatin is well tolerated. However, the observation of cataracts in beagle dogs taking large doses of lovastatin has led the Food and Drug Administration to recommend examination of the lens by slit lamp every 12 months in patients treated with lovastatin. Acute myositis occurs in 0.5% of patients taking this drug [21]. The risk of myositis increases substantially for patients concurrently taking gemfibrozil (5%) or cyclosporine (30%). Rhabdomyolysis with renal failure has occurred. Marked, persistent increases in transaminase levels also occur in 2% of patients taking lovastatin. The most common side effects are flatulence, diarrhea, and sleep disorders. Animal studies using 500 times the maximum human dose have shown teratogenicity; lovastatin is contraindicated during pregnancy. Treatment with lovastatin is begun with 20 mg daily and may be increased to 80 mg daily.

Simvastatin doses range from 10 to 40 mg. It reduces plasma total and LDL cholesterol concentrations by about 30 to 45% and also produces a beneficial and moderate decrease in plasma TG and a small but significant increase in HDL cholesterol [22].

These drugs, though usually well tolerated, should not be the drug of first choice for lowering LDL levels because it has not been associated yet with reduction of coronary artery disease or generated a long track record of safety.

Fish oils [23] containing large amounts of *n*-3 fatty acids are effective in lowering VLDL levels when given in large amounts. However, they tend to raise LDLC levels and depress HDLC levels.

Sometimes patients with severe LDLC levels require therapy with two or three lipid lowering agents to normalize LDL levels. The combination [24] of a bile acid sequestrant with nicotinic acid is synergistic as it pairs one agent that enhance clearance of LDL with another that limits LDL synthesis. This combination showed progression and even led to regression of angiographically assessed atherosclerosis in the CLAS trial [5]. Similarly, concurrent use of a fibrate with a resin can be used in patients with mild hypertriglyceridemia and an elevation of LDLC level.

Pairing a bile acid sequestrant with a HmG CoA reductase inhibitor is particularly synergistic, since it couples two agents that stimulate LDL receptor activity by different means.

Furthermore, the reductase inhibitor limits the compensatory increase in hepatic cholesterol synthesis that occurs when bile acid sequestrants are used alone.

An increased risk of myositis seems to occur when gemfibrozil and lovastatin are used together and caution is urged on this combination. The 3 drug combinations [25] of a bile acid sequestrant, nicotinic acid and a reductase inhibitor can reduce LDL levels and raise HDL levels markedly in patients with severe familial hypercholesterolemia.

Hyperlipemic treatment in patients with renal failure

There is no unanimity on the clinical consequences of the hyperlipemia of the nephrotic syndrome which is characterized by raised total and LDLC with normal or reduced HDLC [26, 27]; in non-nephrotic patients this condition is associated with accelerated atherosclerosis.

Studies demonstrating accelerated atherosclerosis were confounded by inclusion of patients with diabetes mellitus or on steroid treatment, whereas studies which were not demonstrating that complication can be criticized for their inclusion criteria [28, 29].

Hyperlipemia may also be regarded as a pathogenetic factor in the development of focal and segmental glomerulosclerosis [30].

Recent studies [31, 32] have indeed shown that lipid lowering therapy reduced the incidence of focal glomerulosclerosis in animal models. In addition, cholesterol supplementation accelerated the development of focal glomerulosclerosis and aggravated proteinuria in a rat model of the nephrotic syndrome [33]. During the last years, an increasing number of patients with end stage renal disease are being treated by continuous ambulatory peritoneal dialysis (CAPD). Although the CAPD treatment potentially provides several advantages for some patients, one of the major complications associated with this technique, is the development of hyper-lipemia. Between 60 and 80% of the patients develop a hyper TG, while about 30% develop a hypercholesterolemia (increase in TC, LDLC and VLDLC) during CAPD treatment. The available treatments for the management of the secondary hyperlipemia in these patients are limited. This is due to both the lack of a substitute for glucose as osmotic agent, and to the limited efficiency and potential drawbacks of the classical hypolipemic drugs in patients with end stage renal disease.

Also, few controlled studies have been carried out to assess the efficacy of lipid lowering drugs in nephrotic hyperlipemia and most of the drugs do not restore to normal the lipid abnormalities associated with nephrotic syndrome.

Colestipol [33, 34] a bile acid binding resin, has been reported to lower TC and LDLC, but also to raise TG levels. Probucol had moderate effects on total cholesterol and LDLC. It reduced however also HDLC levels, leaving the LDLC/HDLC ratio unchanged. Treatment of nephrotic hyperlipemia with clofibrate [35] has been associated with serious muscle toxicity. Lovastatine [36] and simvastatine [37] two recently introduced HmG CoA reductase inhibitors, induced an important decrease of TC and LDLC in nephrotic patients with hyperlipemia. They are more effective and better tolerated than the resins or clofibrate. Since renal elimination is minimal for the HMG CoA reductase inhibitors, the dosage must not be adjusted in nephrotic patients. The same satisfactory results were obtained in a group of hyperlipemic CAPD patients treated with simvastatin [38].

References

1. Kannel WB, Castelli WP, Gordon T, 1979: Cholesterol in prediction of atherosclerotic disease: New perspectives based on the Framingham Study. Ann Int Med 1986; 90: 85–91.
2. Assmann G, Schulte H, 1986: PROCAM trial, Hedingen, Zurich.
3. The Lipid Research Clinics Coronary Primary Prevention Trial Results, I: Reduction in incidence of coronary heart disease. JAMA 1984: 251: 351–364.
4. The Lipid Research Clinics Coronary Primary Prevention Trial Results, II: The relation of reduction in incidence of coronary heart disease to cholesterol lowering. JAMA 1984: 251: 365–374.
5. Blankenhorn DH, Nessim SA, Johnson RL, Sanmarco ME, Azen SP, Cashin-Hemphill L, 1987: Beneficial effects of combined colestipol-niacin therapy on coronary atherosclerosis and coronary venous bypass grafts. JAMA 257: 3233–40.
6. Frick MH, Elo O, Haapa K, et al., 1987: Helsinki Heart Study: primary-prevention trial with gemfibrozil in middle-aged men with dyslipidemia. N Engl J Med 317: 1237–45.
7. Manninen V, Elo O, Frick MH, et al., 1988: Lipid alterations and decline in the incidence of coronary heart diseases in the Helsinki Heart Study. JAMA 260: 641–51.
8. Expert Panel on Detection, Evaluation, and Treatment of High Blood Cholesterol in Adults, 1988: Report of the National Cholesterol Education Program Expert Panel on Detection, Evaluation, and Treatment of High Blood Cholesterol in Adults. Arch Intern Med 148: 36–9.

9. European Atherosclerosis Society Study Group, 1987: Strategies for the prevention of coronary heart disease. Eur Heart J 8: 77.

10. Brown MS, Goldstein JL, 1986: A receptor-mediated pathway for cholesterol homeostasis. Science 232: 34.

11. Knopp RH, Ginsberg J, Albers JJ, et al., 1985: Contrasting effects of unmodified and time-release forms of niacin on lipoproteins in hyperlipidemic subjects: clues to mechanism of action of niacin. Metabolism 34: 642–50.

12. Grundy SM, Mok HYI, Zech L, Berman M, 1981: Influence of nicotinic acid on metabolism of cholesterol and triglycerides in man. J Lipid Res 22: 24.

13. Canner PL, 1985: Mortality in Coronary Drug Project patients during a nine year posttreatment period. J Am Coll Cardiol 5: 442.

14. Committee of Principal Investigators, 1984: WHO cooperative trial on primary prevention of ischemic heart disease with clofibrate to lower serum cholesterol: final mortality follow-up. Lancet 2: 600–4.

15. Kesäniemi YA, Grundy SM, 1984: Influence of gemfibrozil and clofibrate on the metabolism of cholesterol and plasma triglycerides in man. JAMA 251: 2241.

16. Rössner S, Orö L, 1981: Fenofibrate therapy of hyperlipoproteinemia: a dose-response study and a comparison with clofibrate. Atherosclerosis 38: 273.

17. Fellin R, Martini S, Crepaldi G, Senin U, Mannarino E, Avellone G, Notarbartolo A, Capurso A, D'Agostino C, Montaguti U, Celin D, Descovich GC, Mantovani E, 1981: Multicenter trial with bezafibrate in primary hyperlipidemia. Curr Ther Res 29: 657.

18. Illingworth DR, Olsen GD, Cook SF, Sexton GJ, Wendel HA, Connor WE, 1982: Ciprofibrate in the therapy of type II hypercholesterolemia: a double-blind trial. Atherosclerosis 39: 211.

19. Grundy SM, 1988: HmG CoA reductase inhibitors for treatment of hypercholesterolemia. N Engl J Med 319: 24–32.

20. Deslypere JP, 1989: Comparison between low dose simvastatine and cholestyramine in moderately severe hypercholesterolemia. Acta Cardiol 44: 379–88.

21. Tobert JA, 1988: Rhabdomyolysis in patients receiving lovastatin after cardiac transplant. N Engl J Med 318: 48.

22. Todd P, Goa K, 1990: Simvastatin Drugs 40: 583–607.

23. Phillipson BE, Rothrock DW, Connor WE, Harris WS, Illingworth DR, 1985: Reduction of plasma lipids, lipoproteins, and apoproteins by dietary fish oils in patients with hypertriglyceridemia. N Engl J Med 312: 1210–6.

24. Illingworth DR, 1984: Mevinolin plus colestipol in therapy for severe heterozygous familial hypercholesterolemia. Ann Intern Med 101: 598–604.

25. Malloy MJ, Kane JP, Kunitake ST, Tun P, 1987: Complementarity of colestipol, niacin, and lovastatin in treatment of severe familial hypercholesterolemia. Ann Intern Med 107: 616–23.

26. Appel GB, Blum CB, Chier S, Kunis CL, Appel AS, 1985: The hyperlipidemia of nephrotic syndrome: Relation to plasma albumin concentration, oncotic pressure, and viscosity. N Engl J Med 312: 1544–8.

27. Bernard DB, 1982: Metabolic abnormalities in nephrotic syndrome: pathophysiology and complications. In Brenner BM, Stein JA (eds). Controversies in nephrology, vol 9, the nephrotic syndrome. Churchill Livingstone, New York.

28. Curry RC, Roberts WC, 1977: Status of the coronary arteries in the nephrotic syndrome

(analysis of 20 necropsy patients aged 15 to 35 years to determine if coronary atherosclerosis is accelerated. Am J Med 63: 183–92.

29. Mallick NP, Short CD, 1981: The nephrotic syndrome and ischaemic heart disease. Nephron 27: 54–7.

30. Diamond JR, Karnovsky MJ, 1988: Focal and segmental glomerulosclerosis: analogies to atherosclerosis. Kidney Int 33: 917–24.

31. Kasiske BL, O'Donnell MP, Garvis WJ, Keane WF, 1988: Pharmacologic treatment of hyperlipidemia reduces glomerular injury in rat 5/6 nephrectomy Model of chronic renal failure. Circ Res 62: 367–74.

32. Kasiske BL, O'Donnell MP, Cleary MP, Keane WF, 1988: Treatment of hyperlipidemia reduces glomerular injury in obese Zucker rats. Kidney Int 33: 667–72.

33. Diamond JR, Karnovsky MJ, 1987: Exacerbation of chronic aminonucleoside nephrosis by dietary cholesterol supplementation. Kidney Int 32: 671–7.

34. Valeri A, Gelfand J, Blum C, Appel GB, 1986: Treatment of the hyperlipidemia of the nephrotic syndrome: a controlled trial. Ann J Kidney Dis 8: 388–96.

35. Bridgeman JF, Rosen SM, Thorp JM, 1972: Complications during clofibrate treatment of nephrotic syndrome hyperlipoproteinaemia. Lancet ii: 506.

36. Vega GL, Grundy SM, 1988: Lovastatin therapy in nephrotic hyperlipidemia: Effects on lipoprotein metabolism. Kidney Int 33: 1060–8.

37. Rabelink A, Erhlens D, Koomans H, Mene R, Joles J, 1988: Effects of simvastatin and cholestyramine on lipoprotein profile in hyperlipemia of nephrotic syndrome. Lancet ii: 1335–8.

38. Matthys E, Schurgers B, Lambergts G, Lameire N, Van de Casteele N, Labeur C, Beisiegel U, Rosseneu M, 19XX: Effect of simvastatin treatment on the dyslipoproteinemia in CAPD patients. Submitted.

Index of Subjects

Developments in Nephrology

1. J.S. Cheigh, K.H. Stenzel and A.L. Rubin (eds.): *Manual of Clinical Nephrology of the Rogosin Kidney Center*. 1981   ISBN 90-247-2397-3
2. K.D. Nolph (ed.): *Peritoneal Dialysis*. 1981 ed.: out of print
   3rd revised and enlarged ed. 1988 (not in this series)   ISBN 0-89838-406-0
3. A.B. Gruskin and M.E. Norman (eds.): *Pediatric Nephrology*. 1981
                                                                ISBN 90-247-2514-3
4. O. Schück: *Examination of the Kidney Function*. 1981   ISBN 0-89838-565-2
5. J. Strauss (ed.): *Hypertension, Fluid-electrolytes and Tubulopathies in Pediatric Nephrology*. 1982   ISBN 90-247-2633-6
6. J. Strauss (ed.): *Neonatal Kidney and Fluid-electrolytes*. 1983   ISBN 0-89838-575-X
7. J. Strauss (ed.): *Acute Renal Disorders and Renal Emergencies*. 1984
                                                                ISBN 0-89838-663-2
8. L.J.A. Didio and P.M. Motta (eds.): *Basic, Clinical, and Surgical Nephrology*. 1985
                                                                ISBN 0-89838-698-5
9. E.A. Friedman and C.M. Peterson (eds.): *Diabetic Nephropathy*. Strategy for Therapy. 1985   ISBN 0-89838-735-3
10. R. Dzúrik, B. Lichardus and W. Guder: *Kidney Metabolism and Function*. 1985
                                                                ISBN 0-89838-749-3
11. J. Strauss (ed.): *Homeostasis, Nephrotoxicy, and Renal Anomalies in the Newborn*. 1986   ISBN 0-89838-766-3
12. D.G. Oreopoulos (ed.): *Geriatric Nephrology*. 1986   ISBN 0-89838-781-7
13. E.P. Paganini (ed.): *Acute Continuous Renal Replacement Therapy*. 1986
                                                                ISBN 0-89838-793-0
14. J.S. Cheigh, K.H. Stenzel and A.L. Rubin (eds.): *Hypertension in Kidney Disease*. 1986
                                                                ISBN 0-89838-797-3
15. N. Deane, R.J. Wineman and G.A. Benis (eds.): *Guide to Reprocessing of Hemodialyzers*. 1986   ISBN 0-89838-798-1
16. C. Ponticelli, L. Minetti and G. D'Amico (eds.): *Antiglobulins, Cryoglobulins and Glomerulonephritis*. 1986   ISBN 0-89838-810-4
17. J. Strauss (ed.) with the assistence of L. Strauss: *Persistent Renalgenitourinary Disorders*. 1987   ISBN 0-89838-845-7
18. V.E. Andreucci and A. Dal Canton (eds.): *Diuretics*. Basic, Pharmacological, and Clinical Aspects. 1987   ISBN 0-89838-885-6
19. P.H. Bach and E.H. Lock (eds.): *Nephrotoxicity in the Experimental and Clinical Situation*, Part 1. 1987   ISBN 0-89838-997-1
20. P.H. Bach and E.H. Lock (eds.): *Nephrotoxicity in the Experimental and Clinical Situation*, Part 2. 1987   ISBN 0-89838-980-2
21. S.M. Gore and B.A. Bradley (eds.): *Renal Transplantation*. Sense and Sensitization. 1988   ISBN 0-89838-370-6
22. L. Minetti, G. D'Amico and C. Ponticelli: *The Kidney in Plasma Cell Dyscrasias*. 1988
                                                                ISBN 0-89838-385-4
23. A.S. Lindblad, J.W. Novak and K.D. Nolph (eds.): *Continuous Ambulatory Peritoneal Dialysis in the USA*. Final Report of the National CAPD Registry 1981–1988. 1989
                                                                ISBN 0-7923-0179-X

Developments in Nephrology

Kluwer Academic Publishers – Dordrecht / Boston / London